SLEEP LIKE
THE DRUG

ROSEMARY NICOL lives with four children. She is a *You Need to Know About Osteoporosis* and the best-sellers, *Coping Successfully with Your Irritable Bowel*, *The Irritable Bowel Diet Book* and *The Irritable Bowel Stress Book*. *Sleep Like a Dream – The Drug-Free Way* was inspired by her own experiences in helping her eldest child to get to sleep.

Overcoming Common Problems

A successful and popular series to give you practical help for the emotional and medical problems of everyday life.

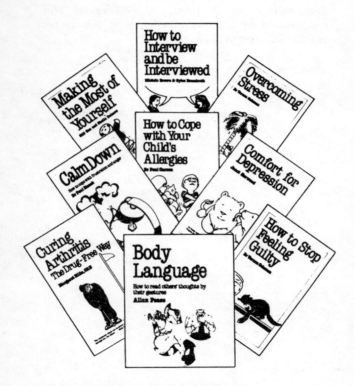

Paperbacks £2·50 to £5·99
Available from all good bookshops

For a complete list of titles write to;
Sheldon Press
SPCK, Marylebone Road, London NW1 4DU

Overcoming Common Problems

SLEEP LIKE A DREAM —
THE DRUG-FREE WAY

Rosemary Nicol

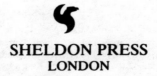

SHELDON PRESS
LONDON

First published in Great Britain in 1988 by
Sheldon Press, SPCK, Marylebone Road, London NW1 4DU

Reprinted with corrections 1991

Third impression 1993

Illustrations by David Barlow

British Library Cataloguing in Publication Data

Nicol, Rosemary
    Sleep Like a Dream — The Drug-Free Way
    1. Man. Sleep
    I. Title   II. Series
    612.821

    ISBN 0–85969–575–1

Typeset by Deltatype Ltd, Ellesmere Port, Cheshire
Printed and bound in Great Britain by
Biddles Ltd, Guildford and King's Lynn

To Katie

I would like to thank my husband David for his loving help, interest and encouragement in the writing of this book. Thanks too to our children, and the many friends, including doctors, who read the manuscript at various stages and offered such helpful advice.

Contents

Introduction   1

1   The Symptoms of Sleeplessness   3

2   The Typical Sufferer   5

3   What Causes Sleeping Problems?   7

4   What is Sleep?   9

5   How Much Sleep do you Need?   12

6   Do you Really Want to Sleep at Night?   14

7   The Helpful Bedroom   16

8   Must you Really Give Up Some of Life's Pleasures?   19

9   Coping with Noise   21

10   Some DOs and DON'Ts   24

11   Learn to Relax   27

12   Food and Drink for a Good Night's Sleep   30

13   Different Types of Insomnia   33

14   Don't Just Lie there — Do Something   38

15   Tranquillisers, Sedatives and Sleeping Pills   42

16   Some Thoughts on Alcohol   47

17   Health Warning — Anger can Ruin your Sleep   50

18 Breathing for Sleeping   54

19 Self-confidence Matters   58

20 Ending the Problem of Sleepless Babies and Children   61

21 Sleep Problems in Older People   69

22 Mental Games   72

23 Baths and Showers   75

24 Alternative Medicine   77

25 Yoga and Meditation   80

26 Commercial Remedies for Sleeping Problems   82

27 And if All Else Fails. . . .   86

    Guide Chart   87

    Further Reading   88

Introduction

With most medical conditions, you visit the doctor, he diagnoses what's wrong with you, and he prescribes medicines which you take according to his instructions. He arranges treatment for you, which you submit to (often at the end of a waiting list). You do all this passively, putting yourself in other people's hands, trusting *they* will make you well again.

But with insomnia *you* can make you well again. You can end this annoying problem when you want to, in your own time, at your own pace, without relying on other people. You can start today, or next week, when you choose, not just when someone is able to give you an appointment.

Why can't you sleep at night? Have you really thought about it, or do you simply toss and turn and curse?

To solve any problem you must first know what's causing it. It may surprise you to know that insomnia is not an illness, but a condition caused by something else; remove the 'something else' and the insomnia should disappear.

Perhaps you can't sleep because your mind is going round and round, or because of noise, or pain, or anxiety, or because you just can't relax, or because of angry feelings. Perhaps your insomnia is caused because you take sleeping pills or alcohol to help you sleep — does that surprise you? Or maybe you have just got into the habit of expecting to be sleepless, or of waking in the night, and you don't know how to alter it.

Although some causes of the problem cannot be easily removed (pain, bereavement, the threat of redundancy, a court case etc.), most of them can, and this book shows you how.

It is designed to be dipped into, not especially to be read through from beginning to end. For this reason, you will notice that some points are repeated in different sections; this is to make sure you don't miss them.

In this book I have collected over 200 different ways to sleep better, from many different sources. Each of them has worked for somebody. So, if you have a sleep problem (or if you have a

1

sleepless baby or young child), then this book is for you.

As you read through the book, don't think 'I'm not going to try that silly idea'; every idea here has already proved helpful to somebody. Only by trying it will you know whether it will work for you.

This book is for people with sleep problems, and is full of ideas and suggestions for them. It is not particularly for those who could sleep falling off a log. So if you are one of the lucky ones who fall asleep the moment your head touches the pillow you may think to yourself, 'This book says don't do this or that, yet I do it and still sleep well'. If the time ever comes when you have difficulty sleeping, you may understand that things which are irrelevant to a good sleeper will become very important to a poor sleeper.

I hope you will find many ideas here to help you, and that after reading this book, your sleep problems will be over.

Rosemary Nicol

1

The Symptoms of Sleeplessness

- Are you tired during the day?
- Does your lack of sleep cause you headaches, irritability and a lack of concentration?
- Do you wake up tired and unrefreshed?
- Do you sleep better away from home than in your own bed?
- Do you always take longer than 30 – 40 minutes to drop off?
- Do you have repeated wakings during the night?
- Do you wake too early and feel unable to get back to sleep?
- Can you only go to sleep with the aid of sleeping tablets or alcohol?

If you answered Yes to most of these questions, then you suffer from insomnia. But don't despair. You are reading this book because it is called *Sleep Like a Dream — The Drug-Free Way* and hopefully by the end of it you will know how to bring your sleep problems to an end.

Many people are convinced that they lie awake sleepless for hours, that they hear the clock strike every hour, and that they 'hardly slept a wink all night'. In reality, the majority of them probably slept most of the night, waking only when the clock chimed or a noisy lorry passed. But they won't believe you when you tell them, and it would take a lengthy scientific experiment involving electrodes attached to the scalp recording different levels of brain-waves to convince them!

You can do your own simpler experiment. For several nights tune the radio to the World Service, or any other radio station which operates throughout the night, and keep it on for, say, 2 hours. Did you really hear every single item in full? Or are there gaps in your memory? Did you pehaps hear the beginning of one item and then the end of the next? After a few nights you may be surprised and relieved that you slept more than you thought.

There are two types of insomnia:

1. *Chronic insomnia* will have lasted for several weeks, perhaps

months, possibly years. Most sufferers fall into one of three groups:

(i) they have difficulty falling asleep when they go to bed;

(ii) they sleep lightly or restlessly, wake up often, and lie awake for hours in the middle of the night;

(iii) they wake very early in the morning and can't get back to sleep.

2. *Transient insomnia* will last from a few nights to 3 – 4 weeks at most. It is usually directly connected with a stressful event such as bereavement, temporary financial problems, a hospital visit, a driving test, exams, a court appearance, an interview or even a wedding. Don't get too worried about it; it should pass quite quickly.

If you spend time lying awake thinking about this new problem of sleeplessness, you will create a viscious circle of sleep problem → worry → more sleep problem. And then when sleep comes it will be stressful, causing you to wake up tired. Transient insomnia badly handled can become chronic insomnia. Don't let it; try some of the ideas in this book before you end up with a serious problem.

2

The Typical Sufferer

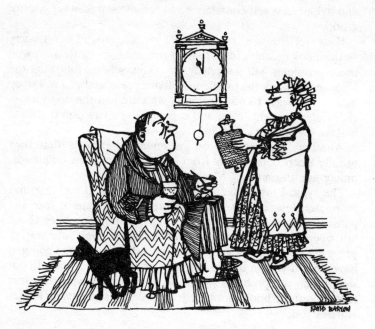

Anyone can suffer from sleeping problems. You may be male or female, young, middle-aged, or elderly, in good or poor health, smoker or non-smoker, it could be you, me, John at work, Peggy next door.

However, some groups of people are more likely to sleep badly than others. Sleeping difficulties are more common among women, especially around the menopause. Women generally sleep more lightly than men, and wake more often during the night. The elderly suffer more than the young, but sleep problems are surprisingly common among young people. Smokers tend to sleep worse than non-smokers, alcoholics worse than teetotallers. And tense, highly-strung people have more sleep problems than calm, tranquil people.

It may or may not cheer you to know that in medical surveys people with sleeping difficulties generally tend to be more worried and depressed, less happy, more sleepy or mentally tired, to have more anxieties about work and personal problems, and to have less self-confidence and self-esteem than the control group.

If you feel you are in one or more of these groups, don't worry — this book contains ideas to help you. Perhaps by sleeping well these problems will disappear, or conversely by following the ideas in this book the problems will disappear and you will sleep better. Anyway, I know sufferers who are just the opposite — cheerful, confident, calm and capable — so you don't want to believe everything you read!

Another characteristic of insomnia sufferers is that they usually sleep better away from home than in their own beds, unlike non-insomniacs. More about this later on.

The typical insomniac dreads yet another bad night, so has more sleeplessness, so worries more, until a state of fear and panic develops, which becomes a self-fulfilling prophecy about not sleeping, and sometimes even a phobia. One sure way to prevent a good night's sleep is worrying that you are not going to have one. If you go to bed in a state of anxiety that you will not sleep, then you probably won't. So read on, following the ideas throughout the book, until the fear of sleepless nights no longer worries you.

3

What Causes Sleeping Problems?

The main causes of insomnia are —

States of mind — anxiety and depression, worry, stress, anger, guilt, bereavement, waiting for something unpleasant (e.g. a court case, an important meeting, notice of redundancy, exams, the results of a medical test — see Chapters 11 and 17).

Your environment — noise (see Chapter 9), discomfort (see Chapter 7), time-zone changes, shiftwork.

Pain — one of the commonest causes of sleeplessness. I would so like to be able to suggest an infallible way of helping you to sleep despite pain, but I regret I can't. Some forms of pain (especially neck, spine, lower back and some joint pains) can be greatly relieved by an osteopath, others by acupuncture. Your doctor may be able to refer you to a pain clinic, where you will be able to discuss all aspects of your particular pain and learn techniques to make it more tolerable. Follow the various breathing exercises, which will help you to relax, and the concentration involved may take your mind off your pain. Also camomile tea and catnip tea with honey have enabled many people to sleep despite pain.

Sleeping pills and tranquillisers are, surprisingly one of the main causes of insomnia; they distort the pattern and quality of sleep, and can also be addictive. Yet 15 per cent of all adults take tranquillisers to help them sleep.

Many medical conditions cause sleep problems, especially heart or breathing problems, stomach and digestive disorders, high blood pressure, arthritis, cancer, kidney failure, Parkinson's disease, starvation (e.g. anorexia nervosa) and some food allergies.

Drugs that can cause sleeplessness include nicotine, caffeine, slimming pills, some contraceptive pills, diuretic or water-reducing drugs (often used for heart trouble or high blood pressure), beta-blockers (also for high blood pressure and

7

anxiety), bronchodilators (for asthma) and stimulants (such as may be prescribed for fatigue or drug-induced sleepiness). But never stop taking drugs prescribed by your doctor without talking to him about it. If you think a prescribed drug may be causing you sleep problems your doctor may be able to change the prescription.

Drugs (the other kind) — heroin, cocaine, cannabis, amphetamines, LSD and other drugs which cause hallucinations — can all cause severe sleep disturbance. It is beyond the scope of this book to recommend methods of drug withdrawal, but obvious sources of help are your doctor, or Narcotics Anonymous, Drughelp, Drugline (listed in many phone books), or your local Citizens Advice Bureau will give you details of help available in complete confidence.

With all these causes, it's not surprising so many people have sleep problems. You are not alone, lying there awake at night. Surveys suggest that half the population suffers from insomnia at some time in their lives, 20 – 35 per cent regularly have difficulty sleeping, and on any one night 15 – 20 per cent are lying sleepless just like you — that's an awful lot of people. With any luck, by the time you have read this book and followed the recommendations you will no longer be one of them.

4

What is Sleep?

What is this thing that occupies about one third of our lives, that we are quite unaware of at the time, and that you are not getting enough of?

If you are really interested in the study of sleep and dreaming, your local library will probably have some interesting books. But if you just want a potted version, then read on.

Sleep is not just one continuous unchanging state of unconsciousness. There are various stages that we pass through during the night, each of which can be identified in experiments by electrodes attached to the scalp recording the levels of brain activity and measured as electrical impulses. These impulses are called 'brain waves', and they vary according to sleep or wakefulness.

As we prepare for sleep, lying in a relaxed wakeful state, our brain produces 'alpha waves'. Then we drift into a transition stage (often called Stage 1), not quite awake, not quite asleep. The mind wanders between fragmented images, and we drift in and out of sleep without realizing it. We may twitch as our muscles start to relax. During this time we are easily awakened, and will insist we have not been asleep.

After about half an hour comes Stage 2, light sleep which takes up more than half our total sleeping time, so is very important. The sleeper will have fragmented thoughts and dreams, and will be awakened by medium levels of noise.

Over the next hour, we drift into the deep sleep of Stage 3, and the even deeper sleep of Stage 4. In Stage 3 the sleeper is quite asleep, completely relaxed but with some movements, and will only be awakened by a loud noise. Dreams are seldom recalled. Stage 4 is the deepest sleep, a state of relatively dreamless oblivion in which the sleeper is difficult to awaken.

During this time of deep sleep (known as non-REM sleep) the heart beats more slowly, blood pressure drops, the breath is slow and regular, and there is no movement. It is thought that during this time growth hormone is produced to restore the body, repair

9

cells, build muscle and supporting tissue, strengthen bones. The feeling of well-being and refreshment that follows sound sleep is probably due at least partly to growth hormone working well.

After about one hour of Stage 4 deep sleep, suddenly the eyelids will start to move rapidly, giving this type of sleep the name of REM (Rapid Eye Movement). Heartbeat and breathing increase, blood pressure rises, we move around in bed. Despite this activity we are still deeply asleep, and difficult to awaken. We are dreaming vividly most of the time, and it is thought that this stage of sleep restores the mind, clears away worries, and maintains brain cells.

A normal night's sleep will consist of cycles of these different levels of sleep. The early part of the night will be mainly deep and light sleep with short bursts of REM sleep. From the small hours of the morning there will be virtually no deep sleep, the same amount of light sleep as before, and much more REM sleep. As getting-up time approaches, we move into Stage 1 transitional sleep, ready to wake up.

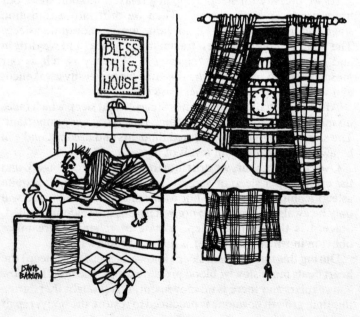

10

Now what use is this information to you if you have problems sleeping?

Firstly, in order to reach the alpha wave stage, you must be in a state of 'relaxed wakefulness'. If you are not relaxed, you will not achieve this stage, as the body cannot support arousal and sleep at the same time, so follow some of the ideas in later chapters to get yourself calm and relaxed by bedtime. By reducing the adrenalin in your body, you give the sleep hormones a chance to work.

Secondly, during Stage 1 sleep (neither quite awake nor quite asleep) you are very easily awakened — a clock chiming, a motorbike going by, people arguing next door, your partner turning over, a breath of wind. You will also find it difficult to know how much of this time you have spent awake and how much asleep. It is extremely common for a poor sleeper to be convinced she was awake for hours, when in fact for much of that time she was lightly asleep, waking only for a few minutes because of a slight disturbance. However honest you are, your mind will deceive you during this transition period. You are probably getting more sleep than you think.

Thirdly, the deep stage of sleep is usually reached within 1–2 hours of going to sleep. So even if you wake up very early in the morning, you have probably had all the deep (Stage 3 & 4 and REM) sleep that you need to restore you.

Fourthly, if you really do get less sleep than you *need* (as compared with what you *want*), it is the deep REM and non-REM sleep that will be increased the next night to compensate. The transition stage will be shortened, and the deep restorative sleep increased. You won't be aware of the different levels, you may think you are still getting only 6 hours or less, but much more of it will be deep sleep, doing you good.

5

How Much Sleep do you Need?

Unfortunately we are the heirs of noble souls like Alfred the Great, and the Hebrew philosopher Maimonides, both of whom said that one-third of our 24 hours (i.e. 8 hours) should be for sleep, and we've been stuck with this idea ever since. Yet only about 60 per cent of us sleep for 7–8 hours, and about one quarter sleep less than 6 hours.

All studies show that most of us get much more sleep than we need, and that short periods of insufficient sleep do not greatly affect us. Despite this, most people feel they must have their 8 hours, and get concerned if they don't.

Constant tiredness during the day is the only sure sign that you are not getting enough sleep. You may sleep for only 6 hours a night or less, but if you are not tired during the day then you do not have insomnia; in your case you may feel happier if you could accept that you need less sleep and use the extra hours constructively (see the final chapter).

If you are a 6-hours-a-night-and-not-tired-in-the-day person, then accept it. Enjoy the extra hours you have. If a young child is awake he will sing, play, talk to himself, look at a book, and be perfectly happy; he doesn't worry about being awake or about not getting a particular number of hours' sleep. You shouldn't either. The answer to your problem may just be to go to bed later.

The average teenager may try and convince you she or he needs 12 hours a night, preferably midnight to midday! But too much sleep or oversleeping for very long periods or just staying in bed too long can produce the same feelings as too little (headache, irritability, drowsiness, etc), and can lead you to believe you have not slept well. If you normally get 10 hours or more, you may feel much better, more alert and energetic, if you reduce your sleep to, say, 7–8 hours.

You cannot judge your own sleep need by comparing it with anyone else's. If your spouse sleeps 8 hours every night, and you sleep only 5 or 6 and are not tired during the day, that doesn't mean you have a problem. After all, we are not all of average build, weight, or shoe size, so why should we be average in our sleep? Some people wake easily, feeling refreshed, early in the morning; others cannot put two thoughts together before 10 o'clock and three cups of coffee.

What matters is the *quality* of your sleep, not the quantity. Six hours of natural restful sleep from which you awake refreshed is much better for you than eight hours of drugged or restless sleep. Learning to relax physically and mentally will improve the quality of your sleep; you will find many helpful ideas further on.

Finally, be tolerant of occasional sleeplessness. When you are *really* short of sleep, nature will make sure you get enough.

6

Do you Really Want to Sleep at Night?

Since insomnia is a problem caused by something else, then if you think you suffer from it (or even if you don't, but you have occasional severe sleep problems), then you have a choice:

EITHER continue your existing life-style unchanged, the same diet, the same alcohol and cigarettes, the same stress and tension, the same attitue to your body, your mind and your spirit — and the same sleepless nights.

OR you can make a few changes: a slightly different diet, less alcohol and cigarettes, some action to reduce tension and anxiety, different routines at bedtime, a new look at yourself — and peaceful tranquil natural sleep. Read on for help with all these things.

One extra thought about you and your insomnia. You may have noticed that many people 'need' their insomnia, like others need 'my headaches', 'my nerves', 'my back' or any other condition. They feel it makes them more interesting. Talking about it makes them feel important. They get sympathy from family, friends, and colleagues at work. They often don't have to do some unpleasant tasks because people know they are tired. They quite enjoy the attention they get. However much they wouldn't want to admit it, they do not really want to be cured. Are you one of these? If so, don't feel guilty about it, but do recognize it and face up to it; don't deceive yourself as well as those around you.

    If you are not prepared to make *any* changes in your life, then the rest of this book is not for you. But if you feel you've had enough of those wakeful nights and tired days, then it just might be worth reading on. Treating sleep problems is not just a matter of taking a pill at bedtime; if your insomnia affects you in an unpleasant way then you must be willing to do things differently, and to make some changes in your life.

14

It is only by commitment to *treating the cause of your problem* that you will achieve a permanent solution.

*　　　*　　　*

So far you have been reading the easy part of the book, nice and descriptive, not requiring you to do anything much except perhaps think 'yes, that's me', or 'no, it isn't'. From now on it gets harder! You will have to *do* things, think a bit, make some changes. But by the end you will know how to beat your sleep problem.

7

The Helpful Bedroom

Your environment and surroundings are important. You should try as far as possible to have a bed that is comfortable, and a room that is dark, quiet and reasonably warm. Unfortunately many people have to make do with unsuitable beds, a noisy environment, a cold room, and a sleeping partner who snores or twitches!

Your bed

A good bed, with a firm sprung base and fairly hard sprung mattress or hard Dunlopillo is your first priority; avoid beds that are lumpy or soft. Always buy the best quality bed you can afford; after all, you spend one third of your life there. In beds as in so many other things you get what you pay for, and a cheap bed may be a waste of money, so go to a specialist bedding shop and spend time choosing the right one.

Don't be embarrassed to lie on the beds — a good shop will expect you to; if they don't want you to, go elsewhere. Try to get advice from someone who has been dealing in beds for a long time — avoid the young salesman who has just got back from a company sales training course!

If you are unable to change the bed (perhaps you are in digs, or you can't afford a new one) place a thick wooden board under the mattress. Get one from a DIY shop or timber merchant, and have it cut to the same size as the frame of your bed.

If your bed is in the middle of the room at present, try having it with one side against a wall; this may make you feel more snug and secure.

It is often suggested that the bed should run north-south, to benefit from the earth's magnetic field. However, I have also seen the suggestion that it should run east-west, so see if one works better for you.

Temperature and bedding

There is no proof that a cold bedroom gives better sleep, though above 75°F/24°C research has shown that sleep quality is reduced, so don't have the bedroom too warm. You do not need to have the window open, it is up to you; try to get a balance so your room is the right temperature, and neither draughty nor stuffy.

Be warm and clean — both contribute to a good night's sleep. When in bed have warm clean feet — wash them every night, and in winter use thick loose-fitting bedsocks if you are cold. Also change to clean sheets and night-clothes at least once a week.

Use a good quality duvet, and air it at least once a week — out of the window on warm sunny days, near a fire or radiator in winter. Or use the drying machines at the launderette on low-to-medium heat. As with beds, you get what you pay for with duvets, so buy the best you can afford, either natural or man-made fillings; 13 tog is ideal unless your room is exceptionally warm. Many people prefer the weight and tight-fitting feeling of blankets, and if you do then use them.

Check that you are not allergic to the material in your duvet, blankets, mattress or pillow; or to the house-dust mite in your bedroom. For instance, do you sneeze or do your eyes water? Many people are allergic to animal products — horsehair, wool, feathers, etc.

In winter wear thick pyjamas or a long thick nightdress, and change to clean ones at least once a week. Even wear a nightcap if your room is cold. Use a hot water bottle, or electric blanket, or thermal underblanket. Try to have night-clothes of natural materials, wool and cotton, rather than synthetic. Surprisingly, many people feel warmer if they sleep naked, so you may like to try that.

Use one pillow or none at all, not more unless advised differently by your doctor.

Light

Some people, especially children, feel comforted by light. If you do, open the curtains slightly, or try a low voltage nightbulb (available from hardware shops).

If you find light disturbing put a soft scarf over your eyes to achieve darkness. Consider changing to thicker, darker curtains.

Noise

Noise is one of the commoner causes of sleeplessness, and all the more annoying because so often we can do nothing to stop it. For some practical suggestions, read Chapter 9, 'Coping with noise'.

Keep a radio by the bed. Speech or music can help you sleep, and can mask outside noise. If possible, invest in a radio with an automatic cut-out which will turn itself off after an hour when, hopefully, you will be asleep; otherwise the radio may wake you later in the night and you will have to turn it off yourself, and may well stay awake. If you do wake in the night turn on the radio, very quietly. Radio 1, Radio 2, World Service and some local and commercial stations are on for much of the night (if you have difficulty sleeping you probably know that already!).

8

Must you Really Give Up
Some of Life's Pleasures?

It seems inevitable in this life that some of the things we like best are bad for us! If you are overweight or have spots you will feel under pressure to give up cakes, buns, sugar, and many of the foods you like most; if you have high blood pressure, diabetes, kidney or liver problems, or indeed any medical problem, you may have to make changes to your diet. So it is with sleep problems. Your heart may sink as you read this list, and obviously it is up to you whether you follow these guidelines, but do at least try — it could make all the difference.

Cut out, or at least cut down on, various stimulants.

- caffeine (which is in tea and coffee), and drink decaffeinated coffee instead of ordinary coffee, and herb or decaffeinated tea, especially from afternoon onwards.
- alcohol — although it may send you to sleep initially, you may wake up after an hour or two and not get back to sleep again. Alcohol taken during the day can cause insomnia at night. Older people are more likely to get insomnia from alcohol than are the young. (Chapter 16 on alcohol, has some helpful ideas.)
- nicotine, (from cigarettes, cigars and pipes) which is a stimulant. Like alcohol, it causes insomnia in older people more than the young. Smokers take longer to get to sleep than non-smokers, and are more wakeful during the night; giving up smoking usually reverses this trend within a few days.
- cola, as in coca-cola, pepsi-cola, etc., which contain stimulants.
- additives in food, especially tartrazine (E102), the yellow colouring that is thought to contribute to hyperactivity in children. Try for a while to eat a diet that is largely additive-free. More and more manufacturers now make food with 'No artificial flavouring, colouring or preservatives', so read the packet before you buy.

19

- avoid junk food and hurried meals. Eat three nutritious meals a day, at regular times, sitting down and feeling relaxed.
- avoid indigestible meals at bedtime. A bowl of cereal with sliced banana will send you to sleep better than king prawn egg foo-yung.
- avoid being seriously over- or under-weight; if in doubt, consult your doctor.
- avoid slimming pills and appetite suppressants unless prescribed by your doctor, as they can cause insomnia.
- many prescribed medicines (such as those for heart disease, high blood pressure, migraine and some contraceptive pills) contain chemicals that can cause sleep disturbance. If you take tablets for these conditions and you have a sleep problem, discuss it with your doctor, who may be able to vary your prescription. If you have to keep taking those tablets, then you may just have to accept that a tendency to insomnia is preferable to your other medical conditions, and learn to live with it.
- finally, at bedtime avoid all arguments, stress and unhappy thoughts. Be forgiving — you'll sleep better. (See Chapter 17, on anger.)

9

Coping with Noise

Noise is a common cause of sleeplessness, and is most disturbing when we are drowsy, such as when falling asleep at night and waking up in the morning. It also causes more annoyance if we feel angry about the cause of it — aircraft, heavy traffic, noisy neighbours, discos, motorbikes, barking dogs etc.

So, as a first step, if you can change your feelings about the noise, which is the subject of this chapter, you may find it less disturbing. If that really doesn't work you could try wax earplugs (from a chemist) and soundproofing double-glazing.

You may be able to lessen some forms of noise yourself by quiet diplomatic action. Many neighbours are genuinely unaware how much their noise disturbs other people, and might respond to a gentle unaggressive suggestion that they turn the TV down, or throw saucepans at each other more quietly. Also some vets are willing to prescribe tablets to reduce a dog's urge to bark incessantly. But keep your cool if you complain to neighbours — do it provocatively and they might take pleasure in making things worse for you. As a very last resort your Environmental Health Officer may be able to help.

Consider two points:

1. Research experiments in sleep laboratories have proved beyond doubt that people can go to sleep and stay asleep despite unbelievably high levels of noise — regular noise, irregular noise, high-pitched noise, low growling noise, piercing noise, monotonous noise, any sort of noise. If they can, so can you.

2. On the whole, children and young people are not disturbed by noise. They seem able to go to sleep and stay asleep despite what you might consider is a dreadful noise. Why? Because the noise doesn't irritate them, doesn't get under their skin. To a child, noisy neighbours and aircraft are not a source of annoyance; nor are motorbikes or discos to teenagers. And because these noises do not annoy them, they do not disturb their sleep.

21

Perhaps you can sleep through thunderstorms, but not through your partner's snores, or through the snores but not through barking dogs, or through the barking dogs but not through the disco, or though the disco but not through your neighbours arguing, or through your neighbours arguing but not through a thunderstorm. And it is almost certain that in houses all around you, people are sleeping peacefully through the very noise that is keeping you awake.

So it is not the level of the noise, or the type of noise, that is keeping you awake, but the way you FEEL about it.

I used to find myself kept awake by windows rattling in the wind. No one else in the house was bothered by this; my husband and four children slept quite peacefully through it all; I was the only one kept awake. If they could sleep through those rattling windows, why couldn't I? Because I expected to wake up and stay awake, and they didn't. I dreaded windy nights in case the windows rattled and I couldn't sleep; they didn't. None of them had any negative feelings at all about rattling windows, so their sleep was not disturbed. (For rattling windows you could read noisy neighbours, discos, aircraft, road works, heavy lorries or whatever keeps *you* awake.)

Having realized it was not the rattling windows but my *attitude* to them that was keeping me awake, I just made myself feel quite calm about it. They were not doing me any actual harm. If they made me wake up that was my fault not theirs. If other people could sleep through the noise so could I, provided I did not let it get on top of me; because the more I worried about it, the less I slept. After all I can sleep through thunderstorms, ghetto blasters, cars backfiring, which shows it is not the *level* of noise that was worrying me, just how I *felt* about that particular noise.

If the noise is caused in some way by other people, try to be forgiving. Getting stewed up is harming you, and having no effect whatever on who or what is causing the noise. Other people around you can sleep through it, and if only you could change your attitude to it, you could sleep too.

So when the noise starts, take some deep slow breaths, relax your body, empty your mind, and convince yourself that tonight the noise will not keep you awake, because you are not angry about it any longer. It worked for me, and it can work for you too.

Finally, try this exercise. Lie in bed on your back, hands resting gently on your abdomen, feeling relaxed all over. Listen to the sounds of your own body — your breathing, heartbeat, digestive rumbles. Notice them, but don't start thinking about them. Next, listen to the sounds in and around your bedroom — your partner breathing, the clock ticking, someone in the next bedroom. Notice the sounds, identify them, but do not start any train of thought about them. Then notice outside sounds — traffic, the wind, birds, people walking by, a dog barking. Again, identify the sounds, but do not allow yourself to think about them.

Now work inwards again — the bedroom sounds, then your body sounds, then out again through bedroom sounds to outside sounds. Follow this sequence for several minutes. It may help you to feel calmer about the sounds that annoy you; you may also notice that while concentrating on one set of sounds, you are less aware of other more annoying ones; and finally by identifying sounds that annoy you, yet not allowing yourself to think about them, you may find you can now go to sleep.

10

Some DOs and DON'Ts

Many insomniacs find they sleep better away from home, or even in the spare room. Why? Because they associate their own bed with sleeplessness. For night after night they lie in that bed wakeful, tense, afraid of not being able to sleep. If this happens to you, you must learn to associate your bed with going to sleep quickly, not with lying awake. So:

- Only go to bed when you are *really* sleepy, not just when the clock says it's bedtime.
- Don't go to bed if you are stressed or unprepared for sleep, or you will lie wakeful.
- Lie down in bed only when you are sleepy, and not before. Read or do breathing exercises until then.
- Don't have arguments in bed; don't associate your bedroom with conflict and worry.
- Use your bed *only* for sleep, and not for watching TV, eating, telephoning, daytime reading, or any other waking activity. (Only sex is excluded from this list.) Thus you learn to associate your bed with sleep, and eventually will go to sleep whenever you are in bed.
- If you can't sleep, get up. Never lie in bed sleepless for more than 30 minutes. Go to another room and do something else until you can't stay awake any longer. Don't fall asleep in that other room, go back to your own bed for that. The chapter called 'Don't just lie there — do something' is full of ideas.

Develop the following habits

- Get up at the same time each morning, even after a bad night, which helps to establish a good sleep/wake pattern and produces better quality sleep.
- Even if you normally rise late, force yourself to rise early; the more hours you have been awake, the quicker you will fall asleep.

- Don't sleep late, even at weekends or on holiday, as this disturbs your sleep pattern, and you will find it harder to go to sleep the following night.
- Establish bedtime habits that give you, say, 7 hours sleep. If you go to sleep too early, don't be surprised if you wake at 5 a.m. If you go to sleep too late, you may find it difficult to wake before 10 a.m. Find a pattern that works for you, perhaps midnight to 7 a.m. You will need to do this in conjunction with other bedtime routines (herb tea, bath, breathing exercises etc., all of which are discussed further on) to make sure you are ready for sleep at the right time.
- Try to be more physically tired than mentally tired when you go to bed.
- Try to eat all your meals in a relaxed way, sitting down, and at regular times; if your digestive system is working overtime you won't sleep well.

DO before bedtime

★ relax for at least an hour. You will not fall asleep if you are upset or excited, so you must calm down first.

★ have a light walk, then a warm (not over-hot) bath.

★ wind down, read, knit, watch TV (but not anything scary or distressing), meditate, listen to music, do some yoga exercises.

★ make sure your body is warm and relaxed, and your mind tranquil.

★ unless you have a serious weight problem, have a bowl of cereal with milk or a warm milky drink or some bread and honey. (See Chapter 12, Food for a good night's sleep.)

★ for your peace of mind do a security check — doors and windows locked, fire out, TV off, cat out etc. Do this thoroughly, but only once.

DON'T before bedtime

★ don't associate your bedroom with conflict and worry.

★ don't solve problems at bedtime.

★ don't have arguments near bedtime.

★ don't have stressful or unhappy thoughts at bedtime — easier said than done though! Try breathing and yoga, and read Chapter 17 on reducing anger.

★ don't take vigorous evening exercise, which produces adrenalin and makes sleep more difficult; instead, exercise in the morning or afternoon.

★ don't fall asleep in front of the television; get into the habit of sleeping only in bed.

★ don't drink too much towards the end of the evening, as a full bladder will probably wake you up.

Many insomniacs, especially women who are tired, nervous or run-down, sleep better and longer at night if they take an afternoon nap. Try to doze for not less than 20 minutes, and not more than about an hour, preferably between about 1 and 3 p.m. If you can't actually sleep, just lie and relax.

This suggestion of a daytime nap may seem to conflict with suggestions elsewhere in the book not to sleep during the day. You must decide which works best for you. If you normally sleep in the day and can't get to sleep at night, then try cutting out the daytime sleep. If you don't normally sleep in the day, try it, and see if it helps. But don't sleep during the evening.

Perhaps you are saying to yourself, 'Where on earth am I going to find time for all this? I've got enough problems fitting everything in as it is.' And therein lies your answer. Too much stress + too much rush = too little sleep. Slow down, think/talk/walk/eat/drive more slowly. And although it seems an arithmetical improbability, the extra time you take doing things *slowly* will give you more time in the day to relax. You don't believe me? Then try it!

11

Learn to Relax

As stress is one of the main causes of insomnia, it follows that if you can reduce the level of stress in your life you should sleep better. So:

- Learn to master the stressful events in your life that are causing you to sleep badly. Stress produces adrenaline, and adrenaline overrides the hormones that normally send you to sleep. Try to sort out your problems (for example in your marriage or at work, debts or anger). If you can't get rid of the problems then try to alter your attitude to them (Chapter 17 on anger, has some good ideas). They are ruining your sleep, and reducing your enjoyment of life. Why should they? Don't let them. If your problems spoil your life then the problems win. Is that what you want?

- Try to keep both mind and body relaxed; if one of them is tense, the other will be too. If mind and body are in a state of harmony you can cope with a lot of stress without it affecting you unduly. But if one of them is ill at ease and out of balance then even a little stress can cause you serious problems, can depress your immune system and make you more prone to illness or disease. Have you noticed how often an illness can be traced back to a time of stress?

- Learn to do things more slowly — eat slowly, walk in a relaxed way, drive calmly and courteously, talk quietly.

- Practise relaxation regularly, say once or twice a day for 10 – 20 minutes, until you know what true relaxation feels like. The more you do it, the easier it will become, and you will find yourself able to achieve peace and serenity at will.

- Plan your day to allow time for leisurely eating. Hurried and inadequate meals will ruin your efforts to relax.

- Try not to worry about the past, or fear for the future. Enjoy today, and make it a good day. At bedtime don't churn over today's events or plan tomorrow's.

- Take regular physical exercise to burn off the cares that get on top of you.

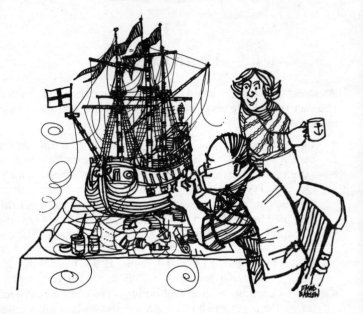

- Develop a non-competitive, creative hobby. Give time to it.
- Even stroking the cat is soothing, and reduces stress and high blood pressure.
- Accept with serenity the things you cannot change. Develop the habit of feeling calm about things that are outside your control. If you can do nothing about them worrying only makes your stress and sleeplessness worse. So try to feel peaceful about the problem until either it is resolved, or you are in a position to influence things yourself.
- An unsatisfactory sexual relationship can be a source of strain. See if you can talk to your partner about any problems, or perhaps your GP or a Marriage Guidance Counsellor could help. Sexual intercourse that is satisfying to both partners induces a good night's sleep. But if one partner finds it unsatisfying for any reason, he or she will probably lie awake unhappy and frustrated. Don't use sex just as a cure for insomnia, as this may be taking advantage of your partner.

28

- Avoid having unrealistic deadlines. Only take on what you can cope with.

- Try to like other people. Treat them as you would like them to treat you.

- Do not take offence. If you do, you can ruin a relationship that you value.

- Don't be a 'busy-busy' person. Do just one thing at a time, and enjoy doing it.

- Breathing exercises can reduce stress, and produce a feeling of calm and well-being (see Chapter 18).

- Meditation induces the alpha brain-waves that normally come before sleep. You may find it helps you (see Chapter 25).

- There are many different forms of relaxation, so why not try one of them — meditation, autogenic therapy, yoga, rhythmic sound repetition, hydrotherapy, and more. If possible get advice on the method from an experienced teacher; as second best, buy or borrow a book on the subject. Or use a relaxation therapy cassette tape (see Chapter 26, Commercial Remedies).

- In times of sudden tension — for example an argument, fear, anger, in traffic jams, waiting for something important or when the children drive you mad — follow this sequence:
    i) take a few deep slow breaths
    ii) drop your shoulders, unclench your hands
    iii) relax your face, jaw and mouth
    iv) lower your voice, and speak more slowly
    v) try and think with compassion and understanding of the situation.

- Do not expect everything instantly. Be willing to wait.

- Give yourself a time of quietness every day.

12

Food and Drink for a
Good Night's Sleep

Have you noticed that many people go to sleep after a heavy meal? Or that slimmers and people suffering from anorexia nervosa often have sleep problems? Could there be a connection?

Follow this simple body chemistry. Many foods contain a substance called tryptophan, which is converted during digestion to an amino acid called L-tryptophan. This circulates in the bloodstream and is subjected to various changes by enzymes. The changed L-tryptophan causes the brain to produce a chemical called serotonin, which is so crucial for sleep it is often called the 'sleep hormone'.

Now, tryptophan in food is not effective in causing the production of this important hormone, serotonin, unless it is taken with carbohydrates, or a combination of carbohydrates and fats, as these liberate the tryptophan to do the job of producing serotonin. Perhaps you can see now how this ties up with the two questions at the start of the chapter — you need carbohydrates or a carbohydrate/fats mix in order to liberate the tryptophan in food to produce serotonin to send you to sleep. Too much and you go out like a light; too little and you can't sleep.

Foods high in tryptophan — milk, eggs, meat, nuts, fish, pulses, cheese (especially Cheddar, gruyere and Swiss).

Foods high in carbohydrates — cakes, sweets, sugar, honey, jam, ice cream, fruit pie, dates, figs, many breakfast cereals, bread, milk, chocolate, potatoes, spaghetti.

Foods high in fats — cream, butter, ice cream, high-fat cheeses, nuts (especially peanuts), fatty meat, saturated margarine, sausages, milk chocolate, peanut butter.

It follows, therefore, that if you can eat the right foods, you should sleep better. Here are three guidelines:–

1.   Eat foods high in tryptophan as often as possible during the day.

2.   If your problem is that you can't get to sleep when you go to bed, eat a meal of high carbohydrates, or carbohydrate/fats combination, two to four hours before bedtime, so the serotonin is released at about bedtime.

3.   If your problem is frequent awakenings, too short sleep, or too light sleep, eat a snack of high carbohydrate, or carbohydrate/fats combination, immediately before going to bed, so the serotonin is released when you might normally be waking in the night. Many people find bread and honey, or mashed banana sandwiches, or a bowl of cereal with milk and sugar and a sliced banana, is ideal.

And in order not to put on weight, restrict most of your carbohydrates and fats to this time, cutting down earlier in the day.

Many women around the menopause have a deficiency of L-tryptophan, detectable by a blood test. This may be one reason why women of this age sometimes develop insomnia.

There may have been comparatively little written on the subject of food for insomnia, but there is no shortage of suggested bedtime drinks. Here are the most common:

★   a warm milky drink at bedtime works very well, perhaps because milk contains generous amounts of tryptophan.

★   most wholefood and healthfood shops sell teas recommended for a good night's sleep, often called Evening Tea or Night Time Tea or Bedtime Tea. They usually contain camomile, and can be wonderful for inducing sleep.

Other teas are:

- camomile tea
- dill tea
- passiflora tea
- catnip tea + honey
- hops and honey
- lemon balm tea

put approx 1 heaped teaspoonful in cup, pour on boiling water, leave to infuse for 4 – 5 minutes, strain and drink.

★ egg nog — heat a cupful of warm milk, add 1 teaspoon of sugar, and either a well-beaten egg or 1 teaspoon of whisky. (If the whisky variation keeps you awake, or causes you to wake during the night, leave it out; see Chapter 16 on alcohol).

★ crush valerian root, infuse in hot water and sip a maximum of 1 cup each night at bedtime.

★ evening primrose root, crushed and infused like valerian.

★ 3 or 4 drops of peppermint essence in a cup of warm water.

★ slice an onion, put the slices in a jug, add boiling water, leave to infuse, strain, and drink warm or tepid.

★ garlic soup, flavoured with vegetable or chicken stock cubes.

★ hot water with lemon and honey.

★ hot red grape juice.

★ hops, infused and strained like onion.

★ 1 part each of hops, pulsatilla, cowslip flowers, and vervain. Pour on boiling water and leave to stand for 20 minutes, stirring frequently, then strain off liquid. Allow 1 oz of the herbs to 1 pint of water. Take one small glass 3 times daily after meals to reduce stress in the day, and so aid sleep at night.

Hops are available from home brewing shops, and the other herbs from wholefood and healthfood shops.

These drinks should be taken about an hour before bedtime. One cup is enough — a large bedtime drink can cause you to wake during the night with a full bladder.

When deciding which of these ideas to try, choose one and stick with it for a week before trying anything else. Don't rush frenetically from one to another; give each one time to work. Having given several a fair chance, you will then know which works best for you.

13

Different Types of Insomnia

There are three main types of insomnia, and this chapter shows you how to cope with each. Some of the ideas are taken from the book *Somniquest*, by Alice Schwartz and Norma Aaron, published by Wildwood House. You may find it helpful to buy or borrow a copy, as it gives detailed step-by-step instructions on how to cope with the different types of insomnia.

1. You have difficulty falling asleep when you go to bed

Unlike other forms of insomnia, this is more common among people in their 20s and 30s, and even younger.

Firstly, don't go to bed until you are quite ready for sleep. If you feel stimulated, lively, wide awake or restless, stay out of bed. If you feel relaxed, calm, or inwardly quiet, either wait a bit longer or go to bed and read or do breathing exercises.

About two to four hours before bedtime have a meal that is high in carbohydrates, or a high carbohydrates and fat combination (see the previous chapter).

Every night when you are in bed say to yourself 'I will fall asleep quickly tonight'. Try to believe it, but even if you don't, your brain will start to work on this new idea by the process of auto-suggestion. Then follow this routine:

If you are still awake after 30 minutes, get out of bed and follow the ideas in Chapter 14, 'Don't Just Lie There — Do Something'. Only go back to bed when you are feeling sleepy, heavy-eyed, or start to nod off.

When you get back into bed, *write down* the time on a piece of paper (don't just make a mental note of it). If you are still awake in ten minutes, write down the time again on that piece of paper. Do the same after another ten minutes. Keep looking at the clock, and do not postpone writing down the time for more than two minutes at the most. If you are still awake, after thirty minutes, get up, occupy yourself as before, and don't go back to bed until you are really sleepy.

Once again, *write down* the time you get back into bed on a piece of paper. And again in ten minutes. And again in another ten minutes. Do not postpone writing down the time for more than two minutes at the most. If you have been methodical about doing this and then you notice that more than ten or twelve minutes have passed and yet you have not written down the time, *then you have been asleep*.

When you first notice those disconnected thoughts, or your muscles start twitching slightly, think to yourself 'I am falling asleep', and you will probably drift into deeper sleep.

If you fall asleep so late at night that you sleep late in the morning, set your alarm for one hour earlier than usual every day for a week, and get up at the new time. However tired you feel during the day, don't smoke, drink coffee, or take stimulants, and don't sleep at all in the day. Do not compensate by going to bed earlier, because you should be going to bed only when you are quite ready for sleep.

After one week set your alarm for one hour earlier still in the morning (that is, two hours earlier than you used to) and get up. Eventually you will be feeling really tired by bedtime, and will go to sleep easily. When you are confident that you can go to sleep within about 20 minutes of going to bed, then you can start to get up a bit later, adding just 15 minutes at a time, and always making sure you can still sleep well at night before getting up later in the morning. Full details of this routine are described in *Somniquest*.

By getting up earlier you increase the length of time you have been awake, and the speed with which you fall asleep is directly related to this; that is why people who have worked long shifts and been awake for a very long time are liable to fall asleep at the wheel of the car without warning. So take care not to drive if you have been awake for an abnormally long time.

Don't regard the weekend as a time to catch up on lost sleep. Keep strictly to the new early getting up time and the same bedtime. If you sleep late on Sunday morning, you won't go to sleep so quickly on Sunday night, and will feel tired on Monday morning.

2. *You sleep so lightly or restlessly that you keep waking up, and lie awake for hours in the middle of the night*

This type of insomnia is more common in people over about 40. If young people have it, it may be linked with depression, and medical help should be sought.

The problem is that you spend too much time in Stage 1 sleep, and not enough time in deep sleep. However, you almost certainly sleep more than you realize, but you only remember when you are awake, not when you are asleep.

At bedtime have a snack that is high in carbohydrates, or a high carbohydrates and fat combination (see Chapter 12, on food.)

When you wake in the night, make a note of the time. If it is say, 3.25 am, resolve to look at the clock in 10 minutes. Do this at 3.35, and again at 3.45. Provided you have noted the time methodically every 10 minutes, then if next time you look there is a gap (perhaps, the time is 4.50 a.m.), then *you have been asleep*. Say to yourself 'I have been asleep, I will go back to sleep again', and recall any disconnected thoughts you had. This will reinforce your expectation of sleep.

If, however, you are still awake after 30 minutes, get up, and follow some of the ideas in 'Don't just lie there — do something'. Don't go back to bed until you can't stay awake a moment longer.

If this waking up in the small hours is a most unusual occurrence, then have a bowl of cereal or a warm milky drink, which should send you to sleep. But if you regularly wake up at this anti-social time, don't eat or drink anything in the middle of the night, for two reasons: a) if you do, you 'reward' your body for waking up, and it will wake you up every night in expectation of this food and drink; and b) if you drink anything, your bladder will send 'getting full' signals to disturb your light sleep.

In order to be so tired at night that you sleep deeply, never sleep during the day, get plenty of vigorous physical exercise preferably before 4 p.m., and get up one hour earlier than usual.

Many night-time awakenings could be due to underlying

anger. Consider if this applies to you, and if it does read the chapter on how to reduce anger.

3. You wake very early in the morning and can't get back to sleep

This is more common among older people, among those who are worried about something particular, and people who are depressed. Depression is a condition which should be taken seriously, and not ignored. Signs of being seriously depressed are: insomnia, especially waking in the middle of the night after a nightmare; loss of interest, energy, and sometimes of appetite; aggression and anti-social behaviour; aches and pains which may or may not have a rational explanation. Some possible causes are:

- Because you sleep badly at night, you often have a long-ish sleep during the day. Then you go to sleep at your normal bedtime, but if you need about 7–8 hours sleep a night, and you use some of that up in the day, then you may well need to sleep less at night, so by the early hours you will have had all the sleep you need.
- Because you wake so early, you are exhausted by 8 or 9 p.m. and cannot stay awake any longer, so you go to bed and fall asleep then. Add 7 or 8 hours sleep, and now it is between 3 and 5 a.m., and you can't sleep any more. So of course the same thing will happen the next night.
- Perhaps, knowing your sleep problems and fearing they will continue (or for other, quite different, reasons), you have a strong drink during the evening . . . maybe several. Then you fall asleep early, perhaps in a chair, and don't wake up until very late at night. You stagger up to bed, probably fall asleep quickly, but then wake at 3 and 4 and 5 a.m., and stay awake.
- Many people who have been taking sleeping tablets for a long time also wake extremely early in the morning.

These are just some of the reasons for waking very early and staying awake. Now here's what you can do about it.

Try to establish a bedtime routine that gives you 7–8 hours sleep at normal hours. So when you feel tired at, say 8 or 9 p.m., force yourself to stay awake. Do the ironing, wash the kitchen, play the piano, sort out some papers, tidy cupboards, clean your workshop, repair the broken whatsit, polish the car . . . anything that requires you to be up-and-doing; whatever you do, don't sit down and relax. (But don't drive, as you may fall asleep at the wheel.) Keep well away from television, and that lovely comfortable armchair. Do everything to stay awake naturally, so don't touch coffee, stimulants or cigarettes. With any luck by about 11 p.m. or midnight you will be well and truly ready for bed, and so should sleep until a respectable waking-up time.

Do this for several nights running to establish a routine. If you do something active during those difficult hours, you also achieve the important aim of being more tired physically than mentally, which possibly you do not usually achieve.

If you normally have a long daytime or early evening sleep, cut it out completely, and do all your sleeping at night-time. For the first few days follow the routine above to keep awake when you would normally fall asleep.

If you usually have one or more strong drinks during the evening, you are not going to like this but I'm afraid you will find it almost impossible to follow this routine unless you can give up alcohol during this period. Why? Because a) the alcohol will make you fall asleep whether you want to or not, b) it will reduce any motivation you may have to stay awake, c) having fallen deeply asleep you will almost certainly wake up after just a few hours and stay awake — because alcohol does that.

Similarly, if you are on stimulants or sedatives (which artificially affect how wakeful or sleepy you feel) you will find this routine difficult to follow unless you can give them up.

*   *   *

Whichever of these three types of insomnia applies to you, don't forget to follow the general bedtime routines — relax for about an hour, have a high carbohydrate/fats snack, a warm bath, a bedtime tea such as camomile, and do some breathing exercises in bed.

14

Don't Just Lie there —
Do Something

Make a rule that you never lie in bed sleepless for more than 30 minutes. As you toss and turn you reinforce the association between bed and sleeplessness. You also take up valuable time which should be spent in deep sleep. So get up, and don't go back to bed until you are really tired.

How will you know when you are really tired? If you feel stimulated, lively, wide awake or restless, stay out of bed. If you feel relaxed, calm, or inwardly quiet, wait a bit longer. If you feel sleepy, heavy-eyed, or start to nod off, go back to bed.

If you are lying sleepless in bed, try some of these ideas:

★ keep your eyes open as long as possible — and then longer (blinking is OK), then inhale with your eyes open, and exhale with them closed. This makes the eyelids feel heavy and can send you to sleep.

★ boredom causes sleep, so read the most incredibly boring book you can find (try your local library), and set yourself a target to read before stopping, perhaps 2 chapters, or 10 pages, or whatever. At the end of each page make yourself remember exactly what that page was about. Or read those pages of your daily or Sunday paper that you find boring.

★ lie on your back with your head flat on the mattress. Relax all your muscles and take a deep slow breath in and out. Then roll your head *very slowly* to one side, keeping your face really relaxed and breathing quietly. When your head has rolled as far as it will go, take a really deep breath in and out. Pause for a moment, then roll your head *very slowly* to the central position, face relaxed, breathing quietly. Pause, and then continue rolling your head to the side, with another deep slow breath at the end. Repeat for as long as you want to, pausing briefly at the central position and at each end. Concentrate on rhythmic breathing and total relaxation.

★ instead of tossing and turning, get out of bed and follow some of the other ideas in this book — a soothing bath, a herb tea, some yoga exercises.

★ practise muscle relaxation — focus on feeling warm and soft in each limb in turn; 'My right leg is soft and relaxed and warm, I am feeling good and at peace.' Do this with each part of your body; do it for one 20-minute session during the day, and again in bed when preparing for sleep. (See Chapter 26 for details of cassette tapes on relaxation)

★ if you are lying sleepless, go to another room and do running-on-the-spot for 5 minutes or more.

★ go to another room, and read a book for 30 minutes standing up.

★ get up and make yourself a cup of camomile tea, or a bread and honey sandwich, or a bowl of cereal with milk. (But if waking up in the middle of the night is a regular occurrence, read p. 35 before doing this.)

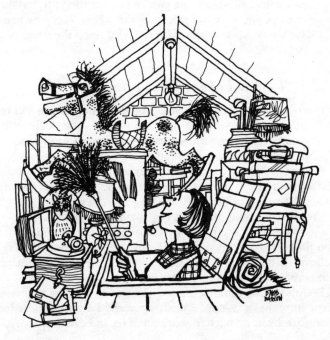

★ instead of trying to sleep, try to stay awake.
★ do something physically tiring, like the ironing, cleaning, sorting out, exercises, etc.
★ find the most uncomfortable position you can, and hold it for as long as possible — and then longer. When you eventually relax, it's a blissful feeling.
★ play mental games (see Chapter 22)
★ do crossword puzzles, logic exercises, or anything that requires your brain to work in short sharp bursts. Reading an exciting book may not be such a good idea if it causes you to stay awake until you finish it.
★ keep awake all night. Choose a day when you have nothing special to do, no work, and especially no driving. Make yourself stay up all the previous night, walk around, be active, but don't go to bed or to sleep. Then spend your day off awake. You may feel very tired during the day, but *don't go to sleep*. Go for a walk, get on with something physically demanding, or something you've been putting off, but don't drive, as you may fall asleep at the wheel. Keep awake all day. By bedtime you will be ready to sleep the sleep of the just!

'I know I'm going to lie awake tonight'

If this is how you feel, then you probably will. As you will read elsewhere in this book, one sure way to lie awake sleepless is to worry about it. So here are some suggestions, some of which are also mentioned in other chapters.

Firstly, follow ideas from throughout the book — have a restful bedtime routine, reduce stress and anger, eat the right foods at the right time, do breathing exercises, make sure your bedroom is working with you not against you, and so on.

Go to bed only when you are quite ready (see Chapter 10). As you lie in bed, say to yourself 'I will sleep well tonight'. Try to believe it, but even if you don't you will be working on your subconscious; so say these words every night.

Follow the routine in Chapter 13 and when you notice you must have been asleep, say to yourself 'I have been asleep; therefore I can go back to sleep', and try to believe it.

As your muscles start to twitch, as disconnected thoughts float across your mind, think 'This means I am falling asleep, so I will soon be asleep'.

If you wake up in the middle of the night, or too early in the morning, say to yourself 'I have been asleep, so I know I can go back to sleep; the only thing that will keep me awake now is if I worry about it, so I am not going to.'

15

Tranquillisers, Sedatives and Sleeping Pills

Do any of these situations apply to you? —

Jane sleeps badly at night, so she is tired during the day, so she takes stimulants to keep awake, so she sleeps badly at night . . . and a habit is formed.

Peter sleeps badly, so he takes sedatives or sleeping tablets. After a while they don't get him to sleep as well as they did, so he increases the dose. Soon even the increased dose doesn't work as well as it did. He has developed a tolerance to them, and his sleep pattern deteriorates.

Anne feels stressed during the day . . . so she can't sleep at night . . . so she takes tranquillisers to relieve the stress . . . so she covers up the real cause of her stress . . . so her stress and sleep problems continue.

Jane, Peter and Anne have also discovered to their distress that if they try to give up their tablets they feel worse than ever.

Do you feel like Jane, Peter or Anne? Surprising as it may seem, regular use of sedatives is a major cause of insomnia and other sleep problems. Sedatives can be helpful if you have *temporary* sleep problems due, say, to a serious personal crisis, but don't get dependent on them. If you use them for more chronic sleeplessness you may get a temporary improvement, but eventually you will have to find a solution that is permanent and satisfying.

Although most doctors only rarely prescribe barbiturates nowadays, even today's sleeping pills, which are much milder, can have undesirable side effects:

- you may get physically dependent on sleeping pills. This means your body gets used to them, and then you need more to produce the same effect.
- you may get psychologically dependent on them. This means

you become afraid to stop taking them in case your insomnia returns.

- sleep-inducing drugs can cause unpleasant side-effects, such as indigestion, skin problems, lowered resistance to infection, poor appetite, high blood pressure, lack of self-confidence, and mental confusion.
- you may wake very early in the morning, and feel tired for much of the day.
- you may feel sluggish and tired when you wake up.
- you may have a 'hangover' feeling, be unable to concentrate properly, make mistakes at work.
- if you drive to work your reactions may be slower, so you are more likely to have an accident.
- sleeping pills also affect the pattern of sleep, depriving you of some of the deep stages that take place during natural sleep. You may dream less, and there may be less opportunity for the body's repair and renewal mechanisms to work; when you give up sleeping pills your body will make up some of the lost REM sleep, so you may have restless sleep, with more dreaming, perhaps even nightmares.
- you may suffer from 'sleep apnoea', a condition in which you stop breathing for several seconds; although usually harmless, it can be quite alarming at the time. It can cause you to wake up hundreds of times during the night as your breathing stops, with the result that you don't get enough sleep, and are exceedingly tired during the day. If you suffer from this condition, get your heart and blood pressure checked, and ask your doctor about a new treatment which involves sleeping with a mask attached to a pump which controls the pressure of the air you breathe. Other ways to overcome this common problem are sleeping on your side instead of your back, and avoiding alcohol, which makes the airways more likely to close. Losing weight also helps, because fat around the neck increases the risk that your airways will close.

Research recently published in America concluded that insomniacs who took sleeping drugs over a long period had as great or greater difficulty in falling asleep or staying asleep, or both, as insomniacs who were not taking sleeping drugs.

Instead of taking tranquillisers and sedatives, use some of the ideas in this book to master the stressful events in your life that are causing you to sleep badly. If you suffer from insomnia which is due to a recognizable cause (stress, anger, pain, etc.) *treat the cause, don't suppress the symptoms*. Unless you learn to cope with the underlying cause, the symptoms will always be there. Sleeping pills do not remove the cause of your sleeplessness, they just cover them up, and make you feel less motivated to solve the underlying problems.

If you are receiving sedatives or tranquillisers from your doctor, talk to him about giving them up. It may take some weeks of gradual withdrawal, and you will need support from him, and from your family, friends and workmates. Be sure to reduce them at a pace you feel you can cope with, because if you try to get off them too quickly you may find yourself back at square one. Don't be tempted to replace dependence on sedatives with dependence on alcohol, or vice versa (see Chapter 16, on alcohol).

Stress and anxiety produce adrenalin, and sleeping pills work by overpowering the adrenalin in your body and enhancing the sleep hormones. When you first try to give up sleeping pills or tranquillisers you will almost certainly get some unpleasant side-effects, possibly starting with a total lack of sleep for two or three nights. This is not unusual, and is caused by the adrenalin which is no longer being suppressed by the pills. You can help overcome this by taking plenty of physical exercise early in the day to use up some of the adrenalin. Eventually nature will make sure you get the sleep you need.

You may also feel more irritable, anxious and depressed until your body adjusts to its normal (pre-sleeping pill) state. As your doctor may have prescribed the pills to control such symptoms in the first place, it is tempting to increase the dose to control the symptoms further. Yet the increased dose will almost certainly make the symptoms worse. So, if you are getting more anxious and miserable despite taking more of the pills, it may be the pills that are causing the problem. Talk to your doctor about cutting down the dose, not increasing it.

If cutting down sleeping pills gives you restless sleep, you may think that therefore you can't sleep without the pills, not realizing that the sleeping pills produced the disturbed sleep first place, and your body is now trying to regain its norma. pattern. So reduce the dose slowly, with your doctor's help, and prepare yourself for several weeks of restless nights.

Many people have a great lack of self-confidence during this difficult time; if you do, read Chapter 19, on self-confidence, which should help you overcome this problem.

As you give up these pills gradually, you will probably continue taking a lower dose for some time. Unless your doctor advises differently, try going to bed with a glass of water and the pills beside you, but only take the pills if you are still awake at about 2 a.m. That way you give your body a chance to fall asleep naturally.

And persevere. Follow the ideas in other chapters (diet, bath, bedtime teas, breathing exercises, learning to relax, etc.) and giving up may be easier than you think.

Finally, to help you decide whether you really do need sleeping pills, here is a true story told by a friend of my husband. He took sleeping pills every night, until, recognizing his dependence and feeling inspired to kick the habit, he decided one night not to take them; but to be on the safe side he left a tablet on his bedside table in case he should need it. Still wide awake at 2 a.m. his resolution failed, and he groped in the dark for the tablet. Instantly he felt better, and before long was fast asleep. Next morning he was surprised to see the sleeping tablet just where he had left it the night before — what he couldn't find was the button waiting to be sewn on!

Useful addresses:

Release
388 Old Street
London EC1V 9LT
tel 071–729 9904

The Phobics Society
4 Cheltenham Road
Chorlton-cum-Hardy
Manchester M21 1QN
tel 061–881 1937

Council for Involuntary Tranquilliser Addiction
Cavendish House
Brighton Road
Waterloo
Liverpool 22 9MG
tel 051–525 2777

Narcotics Anonymous
PO Box 417
London SW10
tel 071–351 6794/6066

ntre
n Lane
Oxley
s
tel 081–428 2483

Families Anonymous
(supports families of those
with a drug problem)
310 Finchley Road
London NW3 7AG
tel 071–834 8121

*Fellowship of Depressives
Anonymous*
(helps people suffering
from depression)
36 Chestnut Avenue
Beverley
Humberside HU17 9QU
tel 0482 860619

Most counties have a council on alcohol and drugs, listed in the phone book under the name of the county (e.g. Somerset Council on Alcohol and Drugs). Despite its rather official-sounding title, it is almost certainly not part of the local authority, but is an organization geared to the needs of individuals and offering a lot of help.

16

Some Thoughts on Alcohol

This is not a lecture on the horrors of the Demon Drink, but as alcohol can cause insomnia, the following thoughts may be useful.

The Health Education Council suggest that in small quantities (no more than 1 glass of wine, or 1 small glass of sherry, or ½ pint of beer or ⅙ gill measure of spirits two or three times a week), alcohol can be beneficial, can aid digestion and reduce stress. But if you regularly drink more than this you may be heading for problems. It may surprise you to know that alcohol is more disruptive to sleep than caffeine — in fact heavy drinking can totally prevent sleep.

Alcohol sends you to sleep — and causes insomnia. You know you find it difficult to get to sleep, so you have a nightcap, sometimes quite a strong one. You go to sleep quite quickly, but as the effect wears off, your body provides extra adrenalin to compensate for the alcohol. Adrenalin overrides sleep hormones, and there you are stuck awake. So you have a nightcap the next night . . .

Alcohol quenches thirst — and makes you thirsty. You feel thirsty, you have an alcoholic drink, it causes your liver and kidneys to work overtime, so you feel thirsty again, so you have another drink . . .

Alcohol can stop your hands shaking — and can cause it. You drink too much, so your hands shake, so you have another drink to stop the shaking . . .

All these problems can become more pronounced from middle age onwards, and especially in the elderly. So why not consider seriously cutting down on alcohol — or even cut it out altogether. Not necessarily 'I will never drink again', but simply 'I will not have a drink today'. It would be worth the effort if you then started to sleep well.

People who regularly drink more than about 5 pints of beer a day, or 10 single whiskies (i.e. ⅙ gill each) run the serious risk of breakdown of family relationships (marital violence, child neglect, separation, divorce), problems at work (poor work performance, risk of accidents, possible loss of job), health problems (liver failure, heart disease, cancer of the digestive tract). Are you heading this way?

Danger signs which indicate you might be heading for alcohol dependence are: a) needing a drink at the same time every day; b) increasing the quantity you drink; c) drinking early in the day; d) drinking secretly and alone; e) feeling you can't sleep without alcohol; f) using alcohol to cope with emotional problems. Be aware of them.

Also, as your doctor may tell you, alcohol can contribute to high blood pressure, especially as you get older, and this can cause insomnia. So *drink less, sleep more*.

Here are just four ideas to help you drink less:

★ Don't drink every day. Have at least 2 or 3 alcohol-free days each week. And don't drink at the same time every day, or while doing the same activity because after a while your body will send 'I want alcohol' messages at that time of day, or during that particular activity.

★ Whenever you feel like an alcoholic drink, drink concentrated apple juice instead, which may reduce your desire for alcohol. Dilute it to about 1 part in 6 with water and drink at least half a pint. You will not get the same beneficial effect from ordinary apple juice in cartons as it is too diluted, so get the concentrate from healthfood and wholefood shops.

★ Don't keep alcohol in the house. If it is there you will probably drink it; if it isn't you can't.

★ When you feel hungry, eat — don't drink. For most people a weight problem would be preferable to an alcohol problem. People who drink quite a lot tend to need a drink when they are hungry, so make sure you eat at regular intervals during the day, preferably wholesome nutritious food, not snacks or junk food. Eat three nutritious meals a day, at regular times, sitting down and feeling relaxed. Don't have a drink just because you feel hungry.

If you feel you may have a drink problem, your local Citizens Advice Bureau will give you details of local organizations and the phone number and first name of a local contact, in strictest confidence. You will not be committing yourself to anything, you needn't even give your name, but it may be nice to talk to someone who understands how you feel.

Useful addresses:

Accept
200 Seagrave Road
London SW6 1RQ
tel 071–381 3155
(for advice, information and counselling)

Al-Anon
61 Great Dover Street
London SE1 4TF
tel 071–403 0888
(offers help and advice to relatives and friends of those with alcohol problems)

Alcohol Concern
305 Grays Inn Road
London WC1X 8QF
tel 071–833 3471
(will give you details of your nearest advice centre)

Alcoholics Anonymous
tel London 071–352 3001   for details
    York 0742–644026   of your
       nearest branch

(or look up details of your nearest branch in your local phone book under 'Alcoholics Anonymous')

17

Health Warning — Anger can Ruin your Sleep

You know it's true, don't you? How many nights have you lain sleepless because you felt angry about something? Your mind churns round and round, you plan revenge, you compose angry letters in your head, you feel resentful, cross and bitter. And you can't get to sleep.

If your sleep problems started after an unhappy experience, or if you often feel depressed, the underlying cause may be anger. Be aware of it.

Perhaps it is unusual for a book on insomnia to include a chapter on reducing anger, but as anger causes many sleepless nights, if you can remove that cause you will sleep better. Some of the ideas which follow may be rather difficult, and I will admit that I find some of them easier to suggest to you than to do in my own life!

- Smile at people as often as possible, whether you know them or not. It is difficult to keep an angry or unpleasant thought in your mind when you are smiling.
- Don't wish evil on the person you feel has wronged you. How would you feel if he were to wish that same evil on you? Really imagine that what you wish would happen to him were to happen to you instead — you wouldn't like it, so don't wish it on him. Your angry thoughts are doing far more harm to you than they are to him.
- Even if someone has done you a wrong, they have almost certainly had some good reason for doing it. Not many people do things solely to spite and hurt someone else. What good motive did that person have for doing what he did? Try and see the situation from his viewpoint, and be forgiving about it.
- However hard it may be, see if you can change your feelings of hate to feelings of liking. The hate is just eating away at you, whereas the feelings of liking will make you feel good. If

you are the sort of person who so often doesn't really like most other people, decide that just for today you are going to like every single person you meet, and you probably will.

- Remember that sentence from the Nun's Prayer — 'Teach me the glorious lesson that occasionally I may be mistaken'.

- Instead of thinking of the person who has wronged you as someone entirely bad, force yourself to dwell on her good points, the kind, generous and caring side of her nature. Even if you have no religious beliefs, try to feel that there is that of God in everyone, even the person you dislike. If you look for the good in people you will find it. Thinking bad of someone causes your muscles to tense, your face to tighten and frown, your eyes to harden; how can you sleep in that state? Thinking well of people makes you feel good in yourself, and calm and tranquil.

- Beat a cushion, imagining the cushion is the person you feel angry about. Don't stop until you have no more anger left.

- When you feel angry, write it all down. Write everything in great detail, even those things you find painful to write. *Then tear it all up*. Don't leave it lying around for someone else to

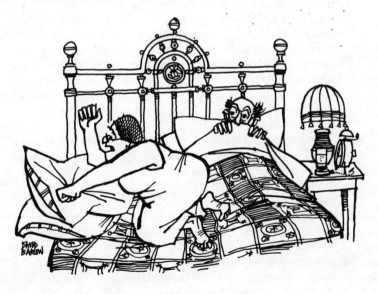

see, or for you to dwell on. When you are angry, the thoughts can completely fill your mind, making it difficult to concentrate on anything else. By writing it down you leave 'space' in your head for more useful thoughts.

- If you feel able, have a reconciliation with the person you feel angry with, either in person or in writing.

- Write 'I forgive X'. And then write down your inner response to saying that, like 'I don't really, because. . . .' Then, again, 'I forgive X', and again write down your further response. Do this until you have nothing more left in you to write. *Then tear it up*. If writing doesn't come easily to you, just say to yourself 'I forgive X', and then say why you don't.

- Forgiveness can reduce anger and lead to better sleep. Perhaps the problem is that you expect X to behave towards you in a certain way, and when he doesn't you feel angry. If you can change your mind about how you feel he should behave towards you, so that you are no longer surprised when he behaves as he does, you will feel better.

- If you can make an effort to feel good about people rather than evil, you will find the bad that is in *you* weakening, and the good that is in *you* raised up.

- People who have difficulty sleeping tend to turn their feelings inwards — anger, aggression, sadness, bitterness, jealousy, fear, guilt. So try and express your feelings in an assertive but non-aggressive way. Listen to what your body is trying to tell you — laugh when you are happy; cry when you are sad; eat when you are hungry and stop when you are full; rest when you are tired; show physical affection to those you love.

- Perhaps you feel that life is treating you badly, that you have had a raw deal, 'Why me? It's just not fair'. Things are not really that bad. Try thinking of the truly awful things that might have happened to you; you only have to read the papers or watch television to see that some people have things happen to them that are so very much worse than what is happening to you. Try and see your own problems as relatively minor compared to theirs. When you hear of something dreadful happening to someone else, hold that person lovingly in your thoughts (even if she or he is unknown to you), and keep your own problems in perspective.

- Next time you are sitting down brooding about someone's behaviour towards you, read these words by Isaac Pennington:

  Our life is love, and peace, and tenderness; and bearing one with another, and forgiving one another, and not laying accusations one against another; but praying one for another, and helping one another up with a tender hand.

Since anger keeps you awake, it follows that if you remove the anger you are also removing one of the obstructions to going to sleep.

All these things are not easy, and are even harder when you are angry or bitter. But work at it, make yourself do it, and it will become easier.

18

Breathing for Sleeping

At various points in this book, I come back to the idea that to improve your sleep at night it is necessary to do various things during the day — the solution to your insomnia is more than just taking a sleeping pill at bedtime. Doing breathing exercises is one step on this path.

Why breathing exercises? Because they can give you energy, they can make you feel calm and relaxed, and they can make you feel good inside yourself.

Your breath is a life-giving force, a source of healing, calm and inner peace. Be aware of it. Use its powers for your well-being. This chapter suggests ways to use your breath when you get up in the morning, during the day, at bedtime and if you are lying sleepless at night.

Develop the habit of deep breathing regularly throughout the day. If you need something to give you a boost of energy or to calm you down *don't* smoke, or have an alcoholic drink, or have a cup of coffee, *but do* breath deeply through your nose.

Do some breathing exercises when you get up, and also find time to do them two or three times during the day for 5–10 minutes at a time. Before you do them, make yourself comfortable and relaxed, and empty your mind of restless worrying thoughts. Give time to them. They can also be very helpful if you are lying wakeful in bed.

Breathing exercise 1

Sit or lie quietly, hands resting in your lap. Breathe deeply and slowly. As you breathe in, think CALM IN, and really visualize a great calm flowing into your body with each incoming breath. As you breathe out, think STRESS OUT, and imagine all the stress, anger, pain and tension leaving your body with each outgoing breath.

Concentrate totally on the breathing, and if your mind wanders bring it gently back to the breathing.

54

Breathing exercise 2 (Alternate Nostril)

Before we start, the Naming of Parts: in order to identify fingers correctly, working outwards from the thumb, they are thumb, index finger, middle finger, ring finger, little finger. So, sit with spine straight, eyes shut and hands relaxed. If you wear glasses it is best to remove them.

1) Place index and middle fingers of right hand on bridge of nose between eyebrows.

2) With ring finger of the same hand close the left nostril. (Reverse instructions if you prefer to use your left hand.)

3) Breathe OUT through right nostril, then breathe IN through right nostril.

4) Lift ring finger slightly and close right nostril with thumb, breathe OUT through left nostril, then IN through left nostril.

5) Lift thumb slightly and repeat from 2) for several minutes, remembering to breath OUT first through each nostril.

It sounds complicated to describe, but once you see how to do it, it is a simple, soothing rhythm. Listen to your breathing. Concentrate on it. If your mind wanders, be aware that it has, and bring it gently back.

Breathing exercise 3 (Solar Plexus)

Do this when you wake up, and at bedtime. Lie flat on the bed. Place hands on your solar plexus, just below the base of the ribs, with fingertips touching. Breathe OUT deeply; pause. Breathe IN slowly through the nose, feel your fingertips separate; pause; breathe OUT slowly, feel your fingertips come together. Continue this slow, calm, deep breathing, and concentrate on your breath. If your mind wanders, be aware of it, and bring it gently back to the breath.

Variation of exercise 3 Instead of pausing, let the inhale and exhale follow each other in one complete circular movement.

Breathing exercise 4

1. Breathe OUT deeply to get rid of stale air.

2. Breathe IN slowly and deeply to count of *two*.
3. Hold breath for a count of *four*.
4. Breathe OUT for a count of *four*.

So you breathe IN *two* — hold *four* — OUT *four*. Do this for two or three minutes, but stop if you feel dizzy. If you have high blood pressure hold your breath for a count of two, not four.

Breathing exercise 5

Open your mouth very slightly, and breathe in and out through your nose and mouth at the same time.

Breathing exercise 6 (Exhale)

1. Breathe IN normally
2. Exhale for as long as you can
3. Breathe IN normally
4. Breathe OUT normally

Continue this sequence for as long as you like.

Each day do one of these exercises when you wake, then two or three times at a quiet moment during the day. After each exercise sit or lie quietly for a few minutes, enjoying the sensation of normal quiet breathing.

If you are lying sleepless in bed, open your eyes as you breathe in, and close them as you breathe out. This makes the eyelids feel heavy, and you will feel sleepy.

If you feel tense during the day, for example in a stressful meeting, or when the children drive you mad, or when you are in heavy rush hour traffic, or during an argument, say no to that cigarette, coffee, or alcoholic drink (all of which may cause sleep problems). Instead, take a few deep, slow breaths, and make a conscious effort to relax, particularly your face, neck, shoulders and hands. You will feel calmer, able to think more clearly.

A word of caution. Breathing exercises can sometimes bring to the surface of your mind thoughts, anger and fears that have been buried for a long time. As a general rule these thoughts are better out than in; be aware of them, but do not let yourself become distressed by them.

If you can practise some of these breathing exercises regularly (say once or twice a day) you will become more peaceful within yourself, and more likely to sleep well.

Meditating

You may remember reading in an earlier chapter that the brain produces different levels of brain-waves, and that alpha waves are the ones produced as we lie in a relaxed wakeful state just before going to sleep. Meditation can produce alpha-waves, so is calming and restful if practised during the day, and can induce sleep if practised at bedtime or if you wake during the night. For a simple way to start, see page 80.

19

Self-confidence Matters

You may recall that in a description of the typical insomniac at the beginning of the book, I mentioned that people with sleeping difficulties tend to lack self-confidence and self-esteem. So, too, do many other people — for example, people who are anxious or depressed, people who are trying to come off tranquillisers and sleeping pills, people going through a difficult patch such as divorce or redundancy.

So here are some ideas to increase your self-confidence. I hope that if you follow them you will also like yourself better, and as a result sleep better.

★ Write out a list of your good points, your skills and talents, the positive parts of your character. Don't be embarrassed to do this, just take delight in being as nice as the list suggests.

★ Walk with your head up and shoulders down, rather than the other way round.

★ Look people in the eye when you speak to them and when they speak to you; this will make you feel more confident.

★ Do something well — anything. When you've done it, recognise that you've done it well, and build on that success.

★ Enjoy being the age you are. Relish its advantages over being older or younger.

★ When you get up in the morning, don't start the new day by stumbling out of bed half-asleep. Spend a few minutes stretching each part of your body in turn, breathing IN as you stretch, and OUT as you relax. Then do one breathing exercise for a few minutes.

★ Have a shower in the morning if you can; the water splashing on your skin is invigorating. Turn it to tepid for a few minutes before you get out, which tones the circulation, improves the metabolic rate, and gives you a good feeling as you start the day.

★ Take regular exercise such as walking, swimming or cycling; or join an evening class or a keep-fit club. You will be surprised how much better you will feel in yourself as you become physically fitter — and how much better you will sleep.

★ Don't get in a rut. Boredom and routine could be your worst enemies. So go to work a different way, eat a different sort of diet, change your hairstyle or the way you dress, watch completely different television programmes, use different shops, change your room around, read different sorts of books, go somewhere else for a holiday. This will stimulate your brain cells, and make you feel good.

★ Get up early, even after a bad night.

★ Have clean freshly-ironed clothes every day, and clean night-clothes and bed linen every week. Feeling dirty and rumpled never did anyone's self-confidence any good.

★ Eat a well-balanced diet, which will make you feel healthy, and therefore good in yourself. A bellyful of stodgy food can make you feel lethargic, bloated and depressed.

★ Are you the type who says, 'If I feel the urge to work I lie down until the feeling wears off!' If so, be active, not sedentary. Gentle exercise is a good cure for fatigue and apathy, so if you feel sluggish get out of that chair and do something physical.

★ As a general rule, for a good night's sleep be more physically tired than mentally tired.

★ Try to cut out (or at least cut down on) alcohol and cigarettes.

★ Go to self-assertiveness classes, where you will learn self-confidence, how to put your point across calmly even if you are nervous or angry, how to meet new people and get on with them, and many such useful skills. Your library or local college should know the nearest ones.

★ Try to feel control over your own life; don't let life (or anyone) run rings round you. Remember winners *make* it happen, losers *let* it happen.

★ Yoga and meditation will increase your feeling of well-being.

★ Breathe deeply into your abdomen. Anxious and shy people tend to hold their breath and to use shallow breathing. So do breathing exercises regularly, especially the alternate nostril method (see p. 55).

★ By buying and reading this book you are working on your problem; accept that as a successful and courageous thing to do.

20

Ending the Problem of Sleepless Babies and Children

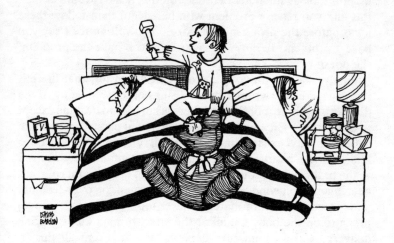

The other chapters in this book are written more for adults (from teenage to old age) than for parents of sleepless children. However this is a problem that can cause such stress in a family that it can lead to baby-battering, divorce, desertion and alcoholism. So I have included quite a large section on how to cope with it, and I hope you find it helpful. If you want to read more, two very helpful books are *Solve Your Child's Sleep Problems* by Dr Richard Ferber, and *Baby and Child* by Penelope Leach.

Sleep problems in children are easier to prevent than to cure. So do your best to prevent them taking hold, but don't despair, most are curable with patience and perseverence. The really important thing is to establish good bedtime habits.

Throughout this chapter I have called the baby 'she' and the child 'he', to avoid being sexist!

Babies

By about three months most healthy full-term infants should sleep through most of the night. I expect you are reading this because yours doesn't!

If your baby is still not sleeping through the night by five or six months look again at her bedtime routine; if she is younger than this and you have a problem with her sleep, then follow these ideas before the problem gets worse. You will notice I say *you* have a problem, because this is true — you have the problem, she doesn't.

Firstly, check with your doctor or health visitor that there is nothing medically wrong that is causing her to sleep badly. If the diagnosis is 'three month colic' there is not a lot to be done except to live with it — it's not your fault and it will pass. Three month colic has always existed, and occurs in all cultures. In China it was known as the 'hundred days crying'. In most infants it rights itself as the brain and nervous system matures. Three month colic has been blamed on wind trapped in the abdomen, on over-feeding, under-feeding, lack of maternal love, too much maternal love, pressure on the baby's skull or the effect of pain killers during delivery, and an immature nervous system. From all this, it would appear that no one really knows! But by following the ideas here make sure that the sleeplessness of three month colic does not become a permanent state when the colic ends.

A very young baby will probably sleep for about 18 hours out of 24, reducing to about 14 hours at night and two daytime sleeps at about 6 months, and about 12 hours at night and one or two daytime sleeps by 18 months to 2 years. Naturally this varies from child to child. But if your baby is awake all evening, goes to bed when you do, and sleeps for a large part of the day or is bad-tempered from lack of night-time sleep, then obviously you have a problem.

Make a clear difference between sleep and wakefulness, so that she soon becomes aware that wakefulness means company, playing and feeding, and sleep means sleep. Don't encourage her to spend ages feeding in a half-awake state. Keep her awake while she feeds, and when the feed is over wrap her up snugly and put her back to sleep in her cot. For night-time sleep make sure the room where she sleeps is quiet and fairly dark. Don't encourage her to drift off to sleep every evening in the living room with lights, television, and above all company, or she will soon become unable to sleep without these things — more of this later.

Develop a good bedtime routine even with a young baby; keep to roughly the same time each night. If you expect your baby to stay up at parties with you, or go to the cinema with you, or be around with your evening visitors, you can't expect her to settle happily to sleep at 6 p.m. tonight because it suits you.

If you want to go out, then get a babysitter; if you can't get one and must take the baby out with you (perhaps to friends or relatives), keep to her usual bedtime routine, and put her to sleep in a quiet room in your friends' or relatives' house. Don't be tempted to get her up to be admired and bounced about. And if your baby has shown signs of sleep problems, try not to alter her routine on holiday, or if you go away for the weekend. It may take a lot of effort to re-establish it.

Ensure her room is warm at night (75°F/24°C). Wrap her up securely; if she kicks her bedclothes off, a one-piece sleepsuit will keep her snugly covered. And make sure that she is warm, well-fed, and cuddled by the time you go to bed yourself.

Having settled her down, leave the door ajar so she can hear household sounds and doesn't feel cut off and alone. Do odd jobs in a nearby room so she can hear you. You are not with her, but you are around, she isn't alone. It isn't a good idea to keep a house with a young baby absolutely silent, with everybody creeping around and talking in whispers. The baby who can only sleep with silence causes a very strained household, and she will wake at the slightest noise, thereby reinforcing the need for silence.

From earliest days, get her used to the background noises of the house, however noisy they are. A baby comes into the world with no pre-conceived ideas of what it will be like, and life will be much easier if she learns to fit in with your ways rather than you having to adapt totally to hers.

Encourage her to have a 'cuddly' — a muslin nappy, old vest, old blanket, piece of cloth, etc — to use at bedtime and to associate with sleep. 'I have my cuddly, therefore I sleep.' If possible, choose for a cuddly something that is replaceable, like an old vest, or muslin nappy, or old piece of soft sheet.

If she cries, go to her quickly, but don't pick her up unless there is obviously something wrong. If you leave her crying it confirms her fear that you are not there and she gets more distressed; and if you pick her up she learns that crying leads to being picked up. Eventually she will learn that you will come if she cries because you are there, but you will not pick her up, take her downstairs, etc.

Personally I do not think it is a good idea to bring her into bed with you at night-time (except perhaps during the brief middle-of-the-night-feed); she will quickly learn that if she cries she will be brought into the warmth, comfort and companionship of your bed, and that habit may be hard to break. I have known 'babies' who still sleep with their parents at the age of seven! I have also known parents whose first child had such terrible sleep problems that they couldn't face the thought of a second child. What a pity that a problem that could have been solved if handled differently resulted in a child being an only child.

Obviously you will have to pick her up if she is crying because it is feed-time, as she will not settle down again if she is hungry, and crying for a long time will only make her more distressed, less likely to feed well, and harder to settle after the feed. But if she has only been fed 1–2 hours ago, and if she fed well, then she is unlikely to be hungry, so don't feed her again. I expect you know babies who run their mothers ragged demanding to be fed every hour, then not feeding much because they are not really hungry, then not sleeping well because they have not fed well, and then waking up soon after to be fed again.

So try and keep her awake during each feed, make sure she takes as much as she needs for her age, and then don't feed her until it is approximately time for the next feed. Try and find a comfortable balance between the old-fashioned strict four-hourly regime, and total demand feeding.

Even a baby can associate sleep with being in a cot in a bedroom, perhaps with a cuddly. To her this combination will come to equal sleep. Now if you always rock or stroke your baby to sleep, or if she always falls asleep in your arms, or feeding, or being driven around in a car, and if you then put her, *already asleep*, into her cot, then when she wakes during the night (as all babies do), this 'going-to-sleep routine' is missing. None of the things she associates with sleep are there. Instead of being rocked, stroked, fed or driven around until she falls asleep again in the night, she finds herself all alone, in a cot, and unable to sleep until you bring back her familiar sleep routine.

So it is important to establish a routine in which she is put in her cot *awake*, with her cuddly if she has one, and that she associates sleep with that cot, in that room, with that cuddly, and learns to fall asleep on her own; so when she wakes in the night (as she will), everything she associates with sleep is there and she will just drop off again.

It has been my experience that in most instances where a baby just will not go to sleep on her own in her cot, this is because she has almost always been lulled to sleep in her mother's or father's arms, and then put back into her cot already asleep. As long as she can wake, look up and see her mother or father there, she will go straight back to sleep; but if she wakes and finds no one there she cannot sleep.

So develop a routine in which your baby learns to fall asleep under the same conditions she would find when she woke during the night — alone and in her cot. Dr Ferber in his book *Solve Your Child's Sleep Problems* describes in detail how to achieve this with a child who will only fall asleep if being rocked, or cuddled, or fed, or with a dummy in her mouth.

Finally, even if your child is now only a baby, read the following section *now* and again in a few months' time. That way you should avoid the problem of sleepless children.

Young children

If your child is no longer a baby, and still has sleep problems, don't despair, it is not too late.

Firstly, read all the previous sections on babies, as your young child's problem may well have been caused by bedtime habits developed when he was a baby, and although you can't put the clock back, it will help if you know why things may have gone wrong.

In general, try not to let bad sleeping habits develop. Keep bedtime at roughly the same time every night, and stick to it. Don't let your toddler decide what time he will go to bed, as this would produce a very haphazard pattern. Learn to say, 'No, you can't stay up to watch that programme, it's bedtime'.

Make bedtime a relaxed, peaceful and enjoyable time of day for both of you — no rows, no boisterous games. Develop a bedtime routine, and keep to it, so he associates that routine with sleep — get him undressed, bath or wash, clean teeth, read him a story in a quiet place, preferably on his bed, and definitely not in front of the television. Give him a loving kiss and cuddle, and settle him into bed with his teddy, doll, cuddly rag, or whatever. Say reassuring words — 'Goodnight, love, sleep well, Mummy's downstairs, see you in the morning' — turn off the light, and leave him.

If he cries, don't let him work himself up into a lather. Go in to him promptly, but don't get involved, don't stay there, don't bring him downstairs with you; just repeat the loving, reassuring words, and go out. Do this as many times as it takes for him to go to sleep. Don't give in! If he associates crying with being brought downstairs, to sit in front of the TV with the rest of the family, you can be sure he will quickly learn!

The idea of a regular routine is that he associates his bed with going to sleep, and not with anything else. So don't put him there to get him out of the way, and definitely not as a punishment; if you do this he will associate his bed with unhappiness and rejection, with crying and fear. If he thinks 'bed = sleep' he will soon fall asleep quickly whenever he is in bed.

He may feel happier with his bedroom door ajar, so he can hear household noises, and a shut door may make him feel shut away from you. I've found children often sleep better if they share a bedroom with a sister or brother. It takes commitment to put a bad sleeper in with a good sleeper, but in my experience the bad sleeper likes the companionship and comfort of his sister or brother, and settles contentedly. Obviously if he disturbs the other one you may have to move him to his own room.

If he wakes distressed and tearful after a bad dream, go into him promptly, don't let him work himself up into a state of distress, give him a loving cuddle, reassure him, and settle him down again. If his bad dreams continue for more than a few nights, try Nelson's homoeopathic remedy Noctura (address in Chapter 26) at bedtime *for a few nights only*, which should improve the quality of his sleep. If the bad dreams still bother him, a practitioner of Bach Flower Remedies or a homoeopath may be able to help, or see your Health Visitor or doctor.

If your child finds it hard to sleep because there is too much light in the room, use heavier curtains, or put dark material over the glass panel above the door.

More likely, your child may not like the dark. Try a low-wattage nightlight, or leave the door slightly ajar, or the curtains open. Follow this simple routine:

1. Go into his room with him after dark, keep the bedroom light on, and open the curtains. It will seem quite dark and black outside.

2. Then turn off his bedroom light, stand by the window with him and enjoy the outside darkness together.

3. Show him how light it is even on a dark night — stars, moon, street lights, lights from other houses, and encourage him to enjoy the darkness as something friendly and non-threatening.

4. Then turn out the landing and other upstairs lights, and enjoy the inside darkness together. Show him it is not really totally dark.

Perhaps give him a cassette recorder in his room, and play tapes of children's stories or songs to lull him to sleep.

Useful organizations:

The National Childbirth Trust has local support groups, through which mothers will help other mothers cope with problems. Your local group will be in the telephone directory under National Childbirth Trust, or your local Citizens Advice Bureau will give you the name of a local contact.

Parents Anonymous (if you are beginning to feel you can't cope) have local branches, many of which are open during the night. Try 071–263 8918, or your local phone book or Citizens' Advice Bureau.

Cry-sis 71 Worsley Road, Manchester, tel 071–404 5011 and *Scottish Cry-sis* 13 Newmans Road, Kirkliston, Edinburgh, tel 031–333 1968 offer help for parents with constantly crying young babies.

An increasing number of local authorities now run Sleep Clinics for babies and their parents. Ask your Health Visitor.

21

Sleep Problems in Older People

Although insomnia becomes more frequent as we get older, sleep *quality* is more important than sleep *quantity*. You may only need 5–6 hours a night, but try to make them peaceful, tranquil hours, and to awake refreshed. And remember that if you need only 5–6 hours sleep in 24 hours, and if you have an afternoon nap, then you have used up some of your sleep need and will probably sleep less at night. Cat-naps are not a sign of reaching your dotage, but are a response to altered patterns in your life; accept them.

In general, older people have less deep refreshing sleep and more light sleep from which they are easily awakened, so they often feel that they have had a wakeful night. Also not only may you have difficulty getting to sleep as you get older, but you may also find it harder to go back to sleep if you wake during the night. You may be woken several times by night-time noises, yet if you go back to sleep quite quickly, and awake refreshed in the morning, you are probably getting enough sleep.

Some causes of insomnia that apply more to older people than younger are:

★ boredom and inactivity (remember, try to be more tired physically than mentally)
★ lack of self-esteem, of any purpose in life; a feeling of being useless
★ pain and discomfort
★ the fact that coffee, smoking and alcohol cause increased sleeplessness as we get older
★ fear of declining health, of losing independence, of the future, of going out at night, of losing family and friends
★ the very common fear of dying while asleep, coupled with the worry 'What will my family do, how will they cope . . ?'

'Sleep and wake' patterns are often altered as you get older because of boredom and inactivity, especially if you have been active. Boredom and inactivity are commonly caused by retire-

69

ment, or if your husband or wife dies and you no longer have a companion to do things with, if someone you have looked after dies or goes into hospital, if you move and leave behind old friends and interests, and if you go into a residential home and don't have to do so much for yourself.

It is not surprising, therefore, that insomnia is extremely common among older people, and unfortunately many overcome the problem with sleeping tablets. But this really should not be necessary. Following the ideas in this book should help you to feel peaceful about these changes in your life, and may reduce any feeling of resentment or bitterness or despair. If you lack self-confidence, or feel bored, or in a rut, read Chapter 19, on self-confidence.

At the risk of repeating what younger people seem to tell their elders and betters ad nauseam, keep active and purposefully occupied. If you feel sluggish and lethargic, try and be active not sedentary. Consider taking up a new hobby, going on outings, developing a new interest; these will give you stimulation and support, a means of filling your days, exercise and friendship. If exercise is difficult for you, do breathing exercises instead.

Eat a balanced diet. Many older people who live alone don't eat well, especially men. If shopping is difficult, perhaps your local Council could provide Meals on Wheels, or a Home Help, or your local branch of the WRVS may be able to help you.

If you are troubled by money worries your local Citizens Advice Bureau may be able to suggest extra forms of cash help. Their service is free and confidential.

Almost everything in the book applies equally well to the elderly as to the young — for example herbal teas to help sleep, a restful bedtime routine, regular unstrenuous exercise, cutting down on alcohol and sedatives, breathing exercises, your attitude to noise and other annoyances in your life, the various mental and physical exercises you can do in bed and at bedtime. So read carefully any chapters that interest you, and follow the various suggestions.

Useful addresses:

Age Concern
Astral House
1268 London Road
London SW16 4EJ
tel 081–679 8000

Help the Aged
St James's Walk
London EC1R 0BE
tel 071–253 0253

REACH (Retired Executives Action Clearing House)
89 Southwark St
London SE1 0HD
tel 071–928 0452
They may be able to find you part-time, expenses-paid work
using your talent and experience to benefit a charity

Carer's National Association
29 Chilworth Mews
London W2 3RG
tel 071–724 7776

22

Mental Games

As with so many other things, there are two schools of thought on the subject of mental games as a cure for insomnia — the DOs and the DON'Ts. The DOs suggest that the mental exercise can send you to sleep, and if they don't then they help you pass the wakeful hours. The DON'Ts say any form of mental stimulation leads to wakefulness, and should be avoided. Try both, and see which works best for you.

If you are a DON'T then ignore this chapter completely, and try some of the other more relaxing ideas instead. If you want to try some mental games here is a selection, all of which have worked for somebody. I have divided them into games involving the manipulation of words, and games that require you to imagine.

Word Games
(to be played in your head, not on paper)

- each night look up a long word in a dictionary, book or newspaper, and see how many 3-letter words you can make from it, then how many 4-letter words, then 5-letter words, and so on.
- spell words and sentences backwards — long words, your address, friends' names, poems, songs, etc.
- think of a song, or a poem, and count how many a's it has, then b's, then c's, and so on.
- list the good things in your life alphabetically: Animals, Brenda, Children, Devoted spouse, Enough money to get by on, Fido, Good health, etc. Think positively about them. If your mind drifts towards your problems, bring it gently back to the good things.
- work your way through the alphabet thinking of a 3-letter word beginning with each letter A through to Z, then a 4-letter word, then a 5-letter word. . . .
- list in alphabetical order places you have visited and

enjoyed, names of people you know and like, animals, books, films, TV or sports people or any subject you find soothing.

- repeat any long piece of poetry or prose (the 23rd Psalm seems to be very popular).

- learn, and recite over and over again, the following poem by Coleridge, which many people find sleep-inducing:

> Oh sleep! it is a gentle thing,
> Beloved from pole to pole!
> To Mary Queen the praise be given!
> She sent the gentle sleep from Heaven,
> That slid into my soul.

(Breathe deeply and evenly while you do this.)

Imagination games

- Imagine in great detail a game you enjoy, and follow every single minute of it. Or recall in great detail a picture, or a walk (see it pace by pace), or a piece of music (note by note). Get really involved in it.

- Imagine that outside there is driving rain, roaring wind, bitter cold and wild animals, while you lie safe and snug in a warm comfortable bed, with a soft pillow, and blankets or a duvet draping gently around you.

- Plan a different house, or new clothes, or car or boat or holiday, or anything pleasant, in great detail (but not anything to do with work or which causes you to feel anxious).

- Try and visualize the word RED written in the colour yellow, and then the word YELLOW written in the colour red, and alternate these two images as many times as you can.

- Visualize the number ONE, and say 'two'; then visualize the number TWO, and say 'one'; alternate these two images several times.

- Recall last night's dream and continue it. Let your mind wander around different dreams you have had.

- Yes, count sheep jumping over a stile! Breathe evenly, counting each one as you exhale.

- 'Visit' a street you know well, or the shops in your High

Street. Imagine yourself at each one in turn, recalling who lives there, or the name of the shop, methodically up one side and down the other.

- Make your mind a complete blank, then imagine a pleasant colour all over, and prevent that colour from taking any shape, just keep it one mass of formless colour. If it does take any shape, bring your mind gently back to the colour. Breathe deeply and slowly all the time.
- Try a mantra (the repetition of one word) — close your eyes and focus your mind on the point at the top of your nose between your eyes. Breathe slowly and deeply. Use one of the following — OMmmm, ONE, PEACE, or any one-syllable word that you find calming.
- To empty your mind of the constant thoughts that so often accompany (or cause?) insomnia, force yourself to make your mind completely empty, thinking of absolutely nothing at all. Do this just for a moment, then gradually try and make that emptiness last for longer. Whenever thoughts come in, be aware of them and throw them away gently to make your mind empty again. With practice you will get better at this.
- Visualize yourself sinking slowly into your bed, each limb and part of your body in turn feeling warm and soft, until you can't feel where your body ends and the bed begins. Do this slowly and imaginatively.

Imaginative words

Here is a selection of 'sleepy' words. Choose one or two that you like the sound of, and let your mind wander imaginatively around them:

lull, somnolence, drowsiness, nodding off, lethargy, heaviness, slumber, dreaming, doze, snooze, dawdle, calm, tranquillity, balm, stillness, hush, unruffled, untroubled, lassitude, leisurely, thoughtful, slowly, pensive, reflective, quietness, warm, serene, comfortable.

23

Baths and Showers

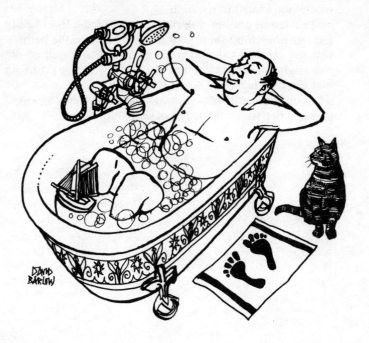

If you have access to a shower as well as a bath, try all these suggestions; otherwise use just the ones you can.

In the morning have a shower (which is invigorating); at bedtime have a bath (which is soothing and relaxing).

Your morning shower (or bath if no shower is available) should be tepid if possible, as this tones the circulation, improves the metabolic rate, and makes you feel good. If tepid sounds too masochistic, start warm (not over-hot) and gradually reduce the temperature until it is tepid by the time you get out.

At bedtime have a comfortably warm (not over-hot) bath with the addition of *one* of the following, which are traditional bath additives for good sleep:

★ boil 1 oz hops (obtainable from home brewing shops) in 1 pint water, strain out the hops, and add the infusion to your bath.

★ add 1 teaspoon camomile (available from health food or wholefood shops) to the bath.

★ make a tea of crushed valerian root (available from health food or wholefood shops), strain, and add it to the bath.

★ suspend crushed valerian roots in muslin or a pair of old clean tights below the hot tap, and let the water pass through it as the bath fills up.

★ add a small quantity of sandalwood oil (from some chemists, perfume departments, or Asian shops) to the bath.

24

Alternative Medicine

Obviously if you have a serious medical problem, it is most important to consult your doctor and get an accurate diagnosis. But sometimes he may be unable to help, and you may want to consider alternative forms of medicine, especially if your problem is chronic or deep-seated.

Many practitioners of alternative medicine are also qualified doctors, but even where they are not they can give extremely valuable help, and often can bring total relief, especially to a long-standing condition, whether physical or emotional. They will treat you as a whole person, not as a collection of symptoms, and will aim to establish harmony and spiritual balance within you.

Response to treatment varies between individuals, but many people quickly notice an improvement in their overall state of health — they may sleep better, feel more relaxed, feel more at ease within themselves, and notice a greater sense of vitality and energy.

Here are some suggestions:

Osteopaths

If you can't sleep because of pain in the neck (including whiplash injury), back (including lower back pain and slipped disc), or shoulders (including a trapped nerve), an osteopath may be able to give more pain relief than your doctor can; he may also be able to solve the problem permanently. Many osteopaths have a better knowledge of bones and joints than some doctors, and many GPs will refer you to an osteopath if you ask. It would probably be a good idea to see your doctor first anyway, in case it is a medical problem that is causing the pain.

Acupuncture

Don't be worried by the thought of needles — they are the thickness of a hair and give little or no discomfort. Acupuncture can help a wide range of conditions, including insomnia and some of the medical problems that cause it, including chronic and severe pain, stress-related disorders, the effects of mental and emotional conflict, as well as many physical illnesses.

Homoeopathy

It works to stimulate the body's power to heal itself, and can be excellent for long-standing chronic conditions, as well as for more acute illnesses. As with most forms of alternative medicine, the homoeopath will consider you as a whole person, not just as a collection of ailments.

Other remedies

There are a variety of other alternative treatments you could try for insomnia. Bach Flower Remedies can give healing for states of mind — anger, jealousy, grief, fear, depression, anxiety, apathy, mental tiredness, irritability, despair, bitterness, intolerance and many more.

The Alexander Technique teaches how to use and move the whole body with maximum balance and co-ordination to increase physical and mental well-being.

You might also want to try herbalism or hypnosis.

Useful addresses:

British Acupuncture Association
34 Alderney Street
London SW1V 4EU
tel 071–834 1012

Homoeopathic Development Foundation
9 Cavendish Square
London W1M 9DD
tel 071–629 3205

General Council and Register of Osteopaths
56 London Road
Reading
tel 0734–576 585

British Holistic Medical Association
179 Gloucester Place
London NW1 6DX
tel 071–262 5299

Society for Teachers of the Alexander Technique
10 London House
Fulham Road
London SW10 9EL
tel 071–351 0828

British Hypnotherapy Association
1 Wythburn Place
London W1H 5WL
tel 071–723 4443

National Institute of Medical Herbalists
9 Palace Gate
Exeter EX1 1JA
tel 0392 426 022

Bach Flower Centre
Mount Vernon
Sotwell
Wallingford
Oxon OX10 0PZ
tel 0491 39489

Institute for Complementary Medicine
21 Portland Place
London W1N 3AF
tel 071–636 9543

25

Yoga and Meditation

Yoga refreshes, invigorates and soothes mind, body and spirit. It can also help many physical and mental conditions including insomnia.

Perhaps you've never done yoga? Don't like the idea of it? Load of Eastern rubbish? You can't see how adopting awkward and unnatural postures during the day can help you sleep at night? Well, if insomnia is a real problem for you, why not make a gigantic leap of faith, and try it just for a few days? Do it in private — no one need know, so you won't feel foolish.

But do it in the right frame of mind — calmly, accepting that what works for millions of other people might work for you. In our Western culture, the physical body is all-important; we largely ignore our mental selves, and almost totally ignore our spiritual selves. Eastern culture believes we are equally mind, body and spirit, and all three must be nurtured; we starve mind and spirit at our peril.

It would not be appropriate for me to describe yoga postures here. Yoga is best explained 'live', so do join a class — most local authorities run them, day or evening. If you really can't, then I recommend the book *Yoga* by Sophy Hoare. It gives good descriptions and photographs of the postures, together with a progressive programme for beginners and more advanced students. There is a list of postures recommended for specific complaints, including insomnia. It is simple and clear, and most suitable for beginners. If you have never done yoga before, some 'deep' books might put you off!

If you would like to try meditating, here is a simple way to start:

Choose a comfortable chair in a quiet room and sit with your back straight, hands on your thighs and feet flat on the floor. Remove glasses if you wear them, and close your eyes. Consciously relax all your muscles, starting with your feet, working up through legs, stomach, hands, shoulders, neck, face, to your head. Relax your tongue, unclench your teeth. Breathe through your nose into your belly, in a normal natural way. Be aware of your breath.

When you are breathing comfortably, say ONE on the exhale, either out loud or to yourself. Then inhale. Do this for 10 – 20 minutes, repeating the word ONE on every exhale. If thoughts come, be aware of them, don't fight them, just try and discard them, concentrating on the repetition of the word ONE, on the rhythmical breathing, and on keeping your muscles relaxed. Then sit quietly for a while, and when you are ready open your eyes.

This method of meditating can also work well if you have trouble getting back to sleep after waking during the night.

26

Commercial Remedies for Sleeping Problems

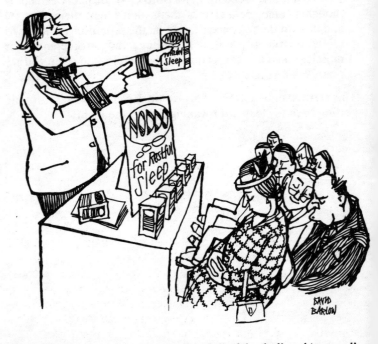

The shelves of health food shops are full of 'herbal' and 'natural' sleeping pills and potions. Some experiments prove they work, some prove they don't. Almost certainly they are not as well researched as conventional drugs, and they may (like any medicines) have side-effects.

Probably this chapter should not be in the book at all, but if you really do feel the need to go out and buy a sleeping remedy, here are some suggestions. As far as I know they are all safe, well-tried, non-habit-forming, and effective, but if you are in any doubt at all ask your doctor, or write to the manufacturers for more information.

Even if research should prove they are medically useless, if they give you a good night's sleep, if you wake refreshed, and if you suffer no side-effects, then surely there is no harm (and possibly some good) in your taking them for short periods.

A word of caution — take any pills as seldom as possible; becoming dependent on herbal or homoeopathic sleeping remedies is perhaps nearly as bad as becoming dependent on conventional sleeping pills. You may not become physically dependent, but you may become psychologically dependent, that is, you may start to think 'I will not be able to go to sleep unless I take my herbal pills'. In any case, you should try first of all to solve the underlying cause of your insomnia before resorting to pills.

It is my personal view that you should not need to take any sleeping remedy for more than a few nights; some manufacturers sell 'a month's supply', but I do feel you should not need this many, and almost certainly not a second month's. If you reach this stage, try the various other suggestions in the book. A good method to follow is '3 on, 3 off' — only take a sleeping pill after 3 bad nights, and stop after 3 good nights.

As you may judge from a short list such as this, herbal, homoeopathic, and alternative sleeping remedies are a multi-million pound business!

I have taken all reasonable steps to check the accuracy of this information, but I'm sure you will understand that I cannot accept responsibility for any changes in products, addresses, or for conditions of use, effectiveness or side-effects. The words in quotation marks are from the manufacturers' literature.

- *Noctura* — 'a homoeopathic remedy for insomnia', from A. Nelson & Co, 5 Endeavour Way, Wimbledon, London SW19 9UH, and from most stockists of homoeopathic remedies.
- *Avena sativa comp.* — 'a natural aid to peaceful relaxation, particularly useful taken at night after a stressful day', from Weleda (UK) Ltd, Heanor Road, Ilkeston, Derbyshire DE7 8DR.
- *Calamite tablets* — 'for sleeplessness due to tension and inability to relax'; also *Pulsatilla compound tablets* — 'when

the body is tired or overwrought', from Frank Roberts (Herbal Dispensaries) Ltd, 91 Newfoundland Road, Bristol BS2 9LT.
- *Waftaway tablets* — 'relieve stress and help promote restful sleep', from Newtons Traditional Remedies, Wast Hills Farm, Wast Hills Lane, Kings Norton, Birmingham B38 9EP.
- *Natu-Rest* — 'a homeopathic remedy for the relief of insomnia', from G.R. Lane Health Products Ltd, Sisson Road, Gloucester.
- *Quiet Night* — 'a herbal remedy for the relief of insomnia', from Health & Heather, Beaver House, Byfleet, Surrey.
- *Passiflora tablets* — 'a herbal remedy for disturbed sleep caused by worry, excitement or overwork', from Potter's (Herbal Supplies) Ltd, Wigan.
- *Valerian compound* — 'a herbal remedy for the relief of insomnia and nervous tension', from Jessup Marketing, 6 Burton Road, Kingston-on-Thames, Surrey.

A selection of cassette tapes designed to promote sleep

Tapes of this kind can be very helpful — in fact I heard of one tape, I forgot which, that took days and days to record because the Sound Engineer kept falling asleep! But don't become dependent on them. Your record shop or library may have a selection.

- ★ *Relaxation for Everyday Living* — 'teaches deep relaxation, relieving tensions and bringing gradual release from drugs and sedatives', from Mary Barfield, 145 Arkwrights, Harlow, Essex CM20 3LZ.
- ★ *Matthew Manning Cassettes*, 39 Abbeygate Street, Bury St. Edmunds, Suffolk IP33 1LW, tel 0284 69502. Tapes for coping with a range of problems.
- ★ Many people find their own voice more soporific than someone else's. If you do, borrow a book on relaxation from the library, and record the relevant parts of it yourself on to a cassette tape. Use a slow calm voice.

COMMERCIAL REMEDIES FOR SLEEPING PROBLEMS

The classified ads section of *Yoga Today, Here's Health*, and similar magazines usually contain several advertisements for cassette tapes to help with stress, sleeplessness, etc. Try your newsagents or library.

27

And if All Else Fails. . . .

Now let us suppose for a minute that none of this has worked. You have tried the drinks, the baths, the exercises, the breathing, the mental games, and all the rest. And tonight, as always, you are still awake. All right then, if you are going to be awake at night, then enjoy it, make the most of it, use those extra hours to good effect.

So when you go to bed, take up with you several quite different books, and your knitting, and those holiday brochures you want to go through, and that report you're working on, and some crossword puzzles, and the gardening catalogues, and last week's Sunday papers, and the list of people you really ought to write letters to. And get on with all these things. As soon as one becomes boring, change to another. Enjoy getting all these things done; think of all mankind fast asleep and not achieving what you are achieving. The night-time noises won't disturb you, because you are not trying to go to sleep. You won't be lying tossing and turning.

If you really do stay awake all night, enjoy what you have accomplished, and feel pleased. More likely, you will find next morning that you fell asleep planning the cabbage patch or writing to Auntie Flo. The less you fear insomnia the less power it will have over you. And when you know you can win, sleep will come like a soft cloud in the night.

Guide Chart

possible causes of sleeplessness	refer to chapter:
alcohol	2, 8, 15, 16
anger	8, 15, 17, 18, 24
babies with sleep problems	20, 26
bedroom, bed and bedding	7
can't relax	11, 15, 17, 18, 24, 25, 26
can't get to sleep once awake	13, 18, 25, 26
children with sleep problems	20, 26
depression	14, 15, 17, 18, 19, 24, 36
difficulty falling asleep	13, 26
drugs	3, 15
expect to have sleep problems	2, 10, 11, 13, 26
keep waking during the night	13, 26
lack of self-confidence	18, 19, 24
light, too much or too little	7
lying awake for hours	10, 13, 14, 26
mind going round and round	11, 14, 15, 17, 18, 24, 25, 26
noise	3, 7, 9
pain	3, 18, 24
sexual problems	11
sleep very lightly	13
sleep better away from home	2, 10
sleeping pills	3, 15, 26
smoking	2, 10, 24
stress, tension	2, 3, 11, 15, 18, 19, 24, 25
tranquillisers	3, 15, 19
unpleasant emotions — anger, hate, jealousy, worry, guilt, anxiety, stress, etc.	3, 8, 9, 10, 11, 15, 17, 18, 25
waking too early	13, 16
worry about not sleeping	2, 10, 15, 18

Further Reading

Borbely, A., *Secrets of Sleep*, Longman, 1986

Bricklin, Mark, *The Practical Encyclopedia of Natural Healing*, Rodale Press Inc., 1976

Chaitow, Leon, *Your Complete Stress-Proofing Programme*, Thorsons, 1983

Culpeper, *English Physician & Complete Herbal*, arr. Mrs C. F. Leyel, Acro, 1961

Dobson, C. B., *Stress — The Hidden Adversary*, MTP Press, 1982

Ferber, Dr Richard, *Solve Your Child's Sleep Problems*, Dorling Kindersley, 1986

Fry, J., (ed.), *The Beecham Manual for Family Practice*, MTP Press, 1982

Hoare, Sophy, *Yoga*, MacDonald Guidelines, 1977

Information kindly supplied by Somerset Council on Alcohol and Drugs

ITV series on Stress, broadcast during 1986

Kales, A. & J., *Evaluation and Treatment of Insomnia*, Oxford University Press, 1984

Leach, Penelope, *Baby and Child*, Michael Joseph, 1977

Luce, G., and Segal, J., *Insomnia*, Longman, 1970

Mitton, Mervyn, *Stress and Tension*, Foulsham, 1984

Nicholson, A., and Marks, J., *Insomnia — A Guide for Medical Practitioners*, MTP Press, 1983

Norfolk, Donald, *Fit For Life*, Hamlyn, 1980

Oswald, I., and Adam, K., *Get A Better Night's Sleep*, Martin Dunitz, 1983

Parkes, J. D., *Sleep and Its Disorders*, Saunders, 1985

Rubinstein, Hilary, *The Complete Insomniac*, Cape, 1974

Schwartz, Alice, and Aaron, Norma, *Somniquest*, Wildwood House, 1980

Tyrer, Dr Peter, *How to Sleep Better*, Sheldon Press, 1978